Praise for So-Called Normal

"From the riveting first line, you'll be taken on an unflinching personal journey with Mark Henick as he saves himself. Learn the backstory to his viral TEDx Talk and be inspired by the heroic act of kindness that made it all possible."
—FRANK WARREN, author of *PostSecret: Extraordinary Confessions from Ordinary Lives*

"In this miraculous story Mark Henick shares a deeply personal tale of growing up in an exceedingly difficult family, his near-suicide and, finally, his journey to an emotionally healthy adult. Compelling, beautifully written and inspiring, Henick's memoir will help you find the light at the end of your own tunnel."
—JAMES MARTIN, SJ, author of *Learning to Pray: A Guide for Everyone*

"Mark Henick gives us the gift of hope by exposing the depth of his pain. In doing so he gives us an understanding of what pain feels like, and when he shares how he found joy in his life, we are left with the unmistakeable feeling that if he can do it, we can do it."
—MICHAEL LANDSBERG, founder of Sick Not Weak and former host of TSN's *Off the Record*

"*So-Called Normal* is a mesmerizing, heart-stopping must-read. I could not put it down! His story is the real thing; I know because I've been there. Even if you have no one in your life who has a mental illness, you must read Mark's book; you'll know much more about mental illness than when you began, and that's important. This book is important!"
—JESSIE CLOSE, author of *Resilience: Two Sisters and a Story of Mental Illness*

"I met Mark Henick two decades ago when he was facing the struggle of living with a mental illness. The story of how Mark took on that challenge and eventually prevailed is important and inspirational reading for anyone who is living with a mental illness or [has] been a family caregiver. I strongly recommend [*So-Called Normal*]."
—SENATOR MICHAEL KIRBY (RETD.), founding chair of the Mental Health Commission of Canada

"*So-Called Normal* is a riveting account of family history, severe depression and the will to find recovery and live with resilience. It's both a moving and powerful story filled with hope. It's a must-read!"

—KEVIN HINES, filmmaker and author of
Cracked, Not Broken: Surviving and Thriving After a Suicide Attempt

"Powerful and real, Henick's story is a stark reminder that we are surrounded by people who struggle each and every day but who 'keep on keeping on.' *So-Called Normal* is a reality check for all, that we still have a long way to go and that advocacy is simply not enough."

—LT. COL. STÉPHANE GRENIER (RETD.), author of
After the War: Surviving PTSD and Changing Mental Health Culture

"*So-Called Normal* is essential reading for anyone dealing with mental health issues. You will come away with a better understanding of what to look for in yourself, your family and friends, and what's at stake. Even when there's despair there can also be help and, ultimately, hope."

—DARRELL BRICKER, author of *Next: Where to Live,*
What to Buy, and Who Will Lead Canada's Future

"This book is a must-read for anyone struggling with, caring for, or trying to better understand mental illness."

—SGT. KEVIN R. BRIGGS (RETD.), California Highway Patrol, author of
Guardian of the Golden Gate: Protecting the Line Between Hope and Despair

"Mark Henick helped save my life one night. This book might save yours."

—WARREN KINSELLA, author of *Web of Hate:*
Inside Canada's Far Right Network

"This is an important and indispensable book about overcoming and triumph, taking us through Henick's wealth of emotions, and each chapter is a precious jewel in the crown of understanding."

—BIF NAKED, author of *I, Bificus: A Memoir*

"This book is a testament to embracing the power within us all and guides the reader as a compass to stay steadfastly committed to their own personal journey, however rocky and jagged that path may be."

—DR. PATRICK SMITH, president and CEO, Centre of Excellence on
Post-Traumatic Stress Disorder and Related Mental Health Conditions

SO-CALLED NORMAL

SO-CALLED NORMAL

A MEMOIR OF FAMILY, DEPRESSION AND RESILIENCE

MARK HENICK

HarperCollins*Publishers*Ltd

Published by HarperCollins Publishers Ltd

First edition

HarperCollins Publishers Ltd
Bay Adelaide Centre, East Tower
22 Adelaide Street West, 41st Floor
Toronto, Ontario, Canada
M5H 4E3

www.harpercollins.ca

Library and Archives Canada Cataloguing in Publication

Title: So-called normal : a memoir of family, depression and resilience / Mark Henick.
Names: Henick, Mark, author.
Identifiers: Canadiana (print) 20200332236 | Canadiana (ebook) 20200332406
ISBN 9781443455039 (softcover) | ISBN 9781443455046 (ebook)
Subjects: LCSH: Henick, Mark. | LCSH: Depressed persons—Canada—Biography.
LCSH: Suicidal behavior—Patients—Canada—Biography. | LCSH: Anxiety disorders—
Patients—Canada—Biography. | LCSH: Depressed persons—Family relationships—Canada.
| LCSH: Suicidal behavior—Patients—Family relationships—Canada. | LCSH: Anxiety
disorders—Patients—Family relationships—Canada. | LCGFT: Autobiographies.
Classification: LCC RC537 .H46 2021 | DDC 616.85/270092—dc23

Printed and bound in the United States of America
LSC/C 9 8 7 6 5 4 3 2 1

This is for you, Mom.
Now I'll let you rest,
so that I may sleep.

Author's Note

*T*HIS STORY IS MY TRUTH. DON'T TAKE THAT TO MEAN that it's anyone else's truth.

I want to be upfront with you about that. That's the whole point of this project, after all. This is my side, my interpretation, my story. On historical facts, dates, places and the like, I tried my best to get them right and to check them as much as possible. I spent hours on research, combing through records and mining other people's memories.

Many of the words or conclusions of doctors, social workers, nurses and other health care providers are quoted or paraphrased from their session notes, which I obtained through the disclosure of my medical records. I also drew information from police and school records. I wove this information in and stitched it together in the way that I felt worked best for my story. I have intentionally changed some people's names and descriptions, where that information is not relevant to retelling my story, to protect their identity. I have also reorganized the details of a small number of events, specifically when they occurred, for the sake of clarity and flow. Some details have almost certainly been unintentionally missed, or edited out to abridge the story. It is also worth noting that I discovered numerous conflicting reports and easily verifiable factual errors throughout these documents, depending on which professional was writing the notes. This validated for me how fragmented my care, and the mental health system more broadly, really was.

You should also be aware that this book will contain triggers for some people. It has descriptions of suicide, including ideations and attempts that I've personally experienced. It also contains descriptions of self-harm, alcohol and drug misuse, bullying and harassment, emotional and sexual abuse, chemical and mechanical psychiatric restraint, domestic violence and police interaction, among other potentially triggering elements. These stories are in here because they happened to me. I've tried to present them realistically, honestly and as part of the much broader and more detailed context of my life.

Part of this journey for me is about learning and respecting people's limits. Discomfort is a healthy, even necessary, part of growth; retraumatizing or vicariously traumatizing yourself is not. If you're not sure how you will react, or if you thought you'd be okay but find yourself passing from discomfort into distress, put the book down. Engage, or discover, your self-care and coping routines, and reach out for help. Do not struggle in silence.

I'm not a doctor. The treatments and interventions that I talk about in these pages, which may or may not have worked for me, may or may not work for you. We may have a lot in common, but your story and your recovery journey are as unique to you as mine are to me. Something that was a disaster for me might end up being the thing that finally works for you. Your journey is yours.

I probably don't know you, but there's a good chance we have had some shared challenges. I've made it through, at least so far, and for as far as I can see into the future. So will you. We didn't come this far to only come this far. If it feels like too much now, trust me, this too shall pass. At the very least, over time, you will learn to struggle well. Years from now, when you least expect it, you may even start to see the gifts that your perseverance left you. Sometimes you don't realize how far you've come until you look back. That's what writing this book taught me.

If you are silent about your pain,
they'll kill you and say you enjoyed it.
ZORA NEALE HURSTON

Prologue

THIS IS THE END.

I'm sure of it. At least, I think I'm sure. I don't want to die. It's just that dying is sort of a non-negotiable part of killing yourself. I have no choice. It feels like nobody can help me, however much they tried, or tried to try. I tried too, for a while. I can't anymore. I can't live like this.

It's nearly midnight. My socks are in my pocket. My feet are cold and naked in my shoes. My heels balance on the chipped concrete edge, while my toes hang out over nothing. I shift my footing and a team of tiny pebbles spills from the side of the bridge. I look down. I watch the pebbles fall as far as I can see them, from my hand-me-down runners to the scraggy ground below. It's probably far enough to do the job, if I can stick the landing as I have visualized so many times. It might be twenty feet down, maybe fifty. I don't know, I'm not good at measurements. I'm not good at a lot of things.

My arms are stretched out along the dull-grey railing that's pressing against my back. My arms are resting on it, not clinging, casually crucified. The four tubular rungs of the railing run horizontally behind me, like a fence that's keeping me outside the land of those who live happily ever after. I don't belong in that place and I never will. The top two rungs curve a little, shifting my centre of gravity. I'm leaning back from the drop, toward the mostly empty road on the bridge that I half crossed to get here. The inward curve was probably meant to stop people from climbing the railing to begin with. I scaled the rungs easily enough, straddled the top, swung my legs over and climbed back down the other side. This isn't my first time here.

I'm calm and tense. My muscles are soft, but my thoughts are tight. I've learned the hard way not to let my body betray my mind's secrets. My fingers are cold and numb, holding me lightly. The railing is wet. It's been a misty Sunday, mid-March, not uncommon on this island. I'm cornered by dirty melting snow all around me, the last of a stubborn winter, splashed into the gutters beside the narrow sidewalk that stretches along the side of the bridge. I think about how much I miss the summer.

This place has been part of the plan for the last few months. The bridge is part of an overpass that connects the two neighbourhoods on either side of the sprawling, shuttered steel plant. There are two worlds beyond my fingertips, to either side of my outstretched arms. In one direction, beyond my right hand, is Whitney Pier. That's where I tried to live, most of the time. Beyond my left hand is the rest of Sydney. I have never been anywhere else and don't know many others who have. Not many people make it out of this place alive. The only way out of the Pier, at least for a kid escaping on foot, is the overpass. At this moment, it certainly feels like the only way out for me.

I study the ground below. There's a long chain-link fence topped with mangled lines of barbed wire. The fence is coated with layers and years of grey paint, but the rust bleeds through anyway. How far out will I need to jump, I wonder, with my peculiar calm rigidity, so I don't land on the fence? The whole point is to end the pain, not add to it. A century of steelmaking has left the ground useless, worn out and toxic. It's dirty and dead down there now, I think. This place understands me. It looks as I feel.

I let my gaze follow the line of the rusty fence. It cuts through the backyards of a row of duplex company houses that border the plant. The second one is my Nana Ag's. It looks small and insignificant from up here. I probably look small and insignificant from down there. Everything feels small, the whole city, yet still I feel smaller. Sydney stands quiet, closed, on the better side of the train tracks that run under the bridge, through Nana Ag's backyard, to the harbour cranes on the horizon in front of me.

Even the bridge itself doesn't really have much purpose these days. The plant has closed and left its waste behind. They'll tear it all down someday, or it will crumble to the ground. The crumbling has been under way for years. For the bridge—and me. That's how things go here. Fall, or be felled.

Now I'm stuck. I can't go back. I won't give them the pleasure. I have to tear it all down. A car passes on the road behind me. It sounds distant and foreign. The driver doesn't see me. Nobody sees me under the incandescent yellow glow of the light post to my left. I used it to steady myself when I climbed over the railing. I didn't want to slip and fall; that wasn't part of the plan. This isn't supposed to be an accident. This is my choice because, as far as I can see, I have no other choices.

I hear another car pass, the sound of tires on wet asphalt, the familiar double thump, the distinctive sound of wheels passing over the exposed steel section connectors that barely hold the old overpass together. A hollow, rhythmic sound—*thump, thump*. For a fleeting moment it breaks the silence around me, it punctures the noise inside me, then it's gone. The noise inside me returns to fill the void, like little underwater explosions.

Thump, thump.

I notice each car that doesn't see me. It's amazing, all we see yet fail to notice.

Thump, thump.

Sure, some people tried to help. Doctors, nurses, parents, priests. Some were nice, some not, most either in the middle or indifferent. I'd become just another hopeless case, a frequent flyer, a lost soul. Abandon hope, all who enter here.

I notice someone over my shoulder. I didn't hear him arrive. He's been talking to me, trying to help. Too bad I'm helpless. The cops are here now too. Beyond my fingertips, in both directions.

I pull my gaze from the unreachable horizon long enough to see that they've barricaded the bridge, that crowds have started to gather. I know they've come to see me fall. I feel nothing. There's nothing to see here. I'm surrounded by people, yet still I'm alone.

There's laughter, somewhere. It's all I can hear, even in the silence, laughter, stabbing me in the head.

Fall, or be felled. Fuck it. I'll tear it all down.

I feel my heart in my chest.

Thump, thump.

My mind is noisy again. There's a lot happening behind me now.

"I tried," I cry aloud. "I tried, I tried, I tried."

Thump, thump.

I can't. I have no choice.

"Jump, you coward!" someone shouts.

Thump, thump.

I let go.

PART ONE

THE SUMMER

Tell me, what else should I have done?
Doesn't everything die at last, and too soon?
Tell me, what is it you plan to do
with your one wild and precious life?

—MARY OLIVER, "THE SUMMER DAY"

CHAPTER 1

I COULD SEE MY GRANDMOTHER'S HOUSE FROM WHERE I stood, on the wrong side of the railing.

I can't remember the names of all Nana Ag's kids. Then again, neither could she. There were seventeen in total, including my mom. Most of those kids had kids of their own, and many of those eventually had kids too. By the time I came along, Nana didn't get too caught up in names. She would rattle off three or four guesses before saying, "Hey you!" She'd point if she meant you. "Who owns you?" she'd ask. Knowing who our parents were at least narrowed the field. It still makes me smile to remember her forgetting our names, long before she forgot us all for good.

The Costigans were a devout Catholic family, Irish via Newfoundland, so that should explain the large family. Nana Ag raised the first half of them, including Papa Mike's five kids from his first wife, in a ramshackle attic apartment above an old movie theatre in the Pier. After the skylight collapsed, raining shards of glass onto one of my uncles in his crib, they decided it was time to find new lodgings. They moved to a little three-bedroom duplex on Railroad Street just before my mom was born. It was a closer walk for Papa to get to work at the plant. He'd bought both sides of the duplex sight unseen but moved his family into only one. He rented out the other side to pay for it. A lot of my memories started on Railroad Street.

My father's parents weren't far behind in the postwar mission to repopulate the earth—or, at least, to populate Sydney. Nana Marg had sixteen kids. The Henick family was Austrian, or German, or Romanian, depending on who you ask, with some more Irish in there because that too was the Cape Breton way. Cape Breton has more fiddlers per capita than anywhere else in the world. The Henicks were nominally Catholic, but nobody would have claimed pious devotion as their excuse for reproducing so extensively. One family story has it that Nana Marg fled to the church down the hill for safety from my shell-shocked and sometimes violent grandfather. She was sent home and told to obey her husband, however many fists or bottles or guns he waved around. That was long before I was born, so I don't remember ever seeing her at mass, or even near a church for that matter. Nobody in the family ever really talks about any of that. Certain things, in some families, are simply unspeakable.

The two big families only occasionally crossed paths in my little hometown. But I was always aware that the two families couldn't have been more different. Conversations with Nana Ag were dotted with attempts to decipher her many Newfoundland idioms—"Y'stay where ya to an I come where ya't!" Nana Marg, on the other hand, amazed us with ever newer and more creative ways of inserting the word "fuck" into places where it otherwise didn't belong—"Dem goddamn cock-fuckin-suckers chargin five fuckin bucks fer a packa smokes!" Smokes were a currency, and a common cause of conflict. She guarded them closely, fishing them out of her bra as needed. As crude as her kids could be—and they could be—they'd never go for them there.

Marg lived up the hill from us, which earned her the name Up Nan, while Agnes lived down the hill, and therefore became Down Nan. We lived somewhere in the middle, between the two houses that seemed like two different worlds, but it was all relative. They reigned over their respective queendoms, one with fury and the other with grace. They were loved and they were needed, each in her own way, by the community of people they'd raised.

For all their differences, they shared a place that had seen a lot of change. It was a different time, when they were raising their families in Sydney. The city, the whole island in fact, was booming. People came from everywhere, by boat over the open ocean and from the seemingly distant Mainland by a narrow, then-busy, causeway. The steel plant and all the industries that grew to support it gave people purpose, meaning, a living wage for an honest day's work. With so many Irish immigrants, heartbreak was a common expectation. Life is hard, that's just the way it is. Everyone here knew that.

By the time I was born, much of the town's glory was gone. So too was the booming industry, the work and wages, the honesty. Many families remained, however. Most did. Where else would they go? This was their home. The plant was mostly still standing, at least until the long-drawn-out efforts to find a buyer dried up. When the six big smokestacks that towered over the tar ponds came down with a crash of dynamite, we watched from the chain-link perimeter fence that cut through the backyard of Nana Ag's duplex next door. The explosion echoed as far as the Cold War radar base atop Blueberry Hill, just behind Nana Marg's house.

One place that remained constant was Holy Redeemer. It was a hundred-year-old red brick church, with a tall, square bell tower, easily visible from the big picture windows in our house up on Lingan Road. Nana Ag and Papa Mike had their children baptized there, instilling in them a lifetime devotion, even after Papa stopped going following the Second Vatican Council. "I don't understand," he said, "how men can just change something that God created."

Papa Mike married Nana Ag at Holy Redeemer, according to the white-glazed decorative plate that hung permanently above their kitchen table. They had a lot of little things like that hanging around the house. We mostly weren't the chapter-and-verse type of Catholics. Still, many in the family could recite the familiar verses, probably thanks to Nana Ag's walls. It was common to find passages inscribed on a piece of wood or porcelain throughout her house and mounted in the homes of all the Costigans. The Sermon on the Mount was popular: the Beatitudes—*Blessed are the poor in spirit, blessed are they who mourn, blessed are the peacemakers*, et cetera—and the Parable of the Wise and Foolish Builders, who built their houses on rock and sand respectively. A large print of the less scriptural Footprints in the Sand story greeted all who entered Nana Ag's front door. It's the tale of a man who dreamt that he walked along a beach with the Lord, reflecting on his life. "During your times of trial and suffering, when you see only one set of footprints," the Lord tells him, "it was then that I carried you."

The Costigans prayed the rosary together, on their knees on the kitchen floor, every Saturday night. Every Sunday morning, rain or shine, they shepherded their herd up Victoria Road to attend mass. They filled the entire first two rows of pews. So central was this place in the life of our family, and the lives of so many other families in Whitney Pier at the time, that the church had to place the pews uncomfortably close together to accommodate the crowds. While it wasn't a problem for most of my mother's vertically challenged family, the lack of space made it practically impossible for anyone over five foot eight to kneel piously upright with a straight back, hips locked, and knees at a ninety-degree angle. The rest of us adopted a sort of seated slouch-kneel instead, perched at the edge of the seat, so that our feet wouldn't hit the knees of the person kneeling in the pew behind us. That's one theory as to why the much taller Henick family were a rarer presence at church each week. Piety is hard when the environment doesn't support it.

Mom continued with family tradition by getting married at Holy Redeemer too, as was expected of her. My dad was the delivery boy for Simon David's grocery store. He brought the groceries to the Costigan house on credit after Papa Mike started drinking away his paycheques. By the time they got married, the Cape Breton decline was already well under way. The girls' school that my mom had attended and the boys' school that Dad nearly finished before dropping out were both long gone. The two junior high schools were gone as well, and the days were numbered for the other Catholic-run facilities across town: the high school, the nursing school, the convent, the two community halls and the hospital. The Catholic Church once had a powerful monopoly in Sydney, but even they couldn't fight the current of change.

Holy Redeemer itself endured, however. Mom cried there for years whenever "Amazing Grace" was sung, after her father died one Halloween morning. He was talking to Nana Ag at their kitchen table, the beating heart of their home, and then suddenly his wasn't. "Amazing Grace" was sung at his funeral. Mom was twenty-nine, a few years married, with a little girl and a newborn boy and a promising new career. When I came along about two years later, Mom willingly fulfilled her obligation to tradition, to expectation, by having all three of her kids baptized at Holy Redeemer.

My mom brought us to church every Sunday for as long as she could. I ended up going to church for a lot longer than my sister, Krista, or my brother, Raymond. Krista never really liked church and was never shy to say so. Raymond went for a while, when we were little, but never seemed to learn how to sit in one place for long, so he stopped going too. I, on the other hand, liked the predictability of the mass, how I always knew what to expect there. I can't be sure, but I think that's what my mom liked about it too in the years after her father's death, and then later as her marriage and everything else around us began to crumble. There's a feeling of safety in predictability.

My mother became a nurse not long after she married my dad. The hours were long, gruelling and often unpredictable. My sister was usually left to care for me and my brother, and there are times when she was the parent I remember most. My dad spent all of his time in the garage he'd built in Nana Marg's yard. His dad had been a mechanic too, in the war. His name was Walter, but everyone called him Tom, like his own father, and his father before that. I never really knew if I was supposed to call him Papa Tom or something else, because nobody talked about him, about his death least of all. Tom died when Dad was barely a teenager. Family rumours—rumours being something at which the Henick family was especially proficient—held that he died on the stairs in their house. He was characteristically drunk and either suffered a heart attack or took a fall. Nana Marg said that she "danced a jig" on the day he died. She could give as good as she got. She had toughened with time, and necessity.

Still, Dad followed in at least some of his father's footsteps. Tradition is like gravity: it'll pull you down the expected path unless you evolve, or invent, some way to fight it. My father had built a small but successful business painting and repairing cars. He built a two-bay garage in Nana Marg's yard, at the top of Brooks Street. He painted *HENICK'S AUTO BODY* on the roof for all down the hill to see, but he accidentally painted the *N* backwards. He decided to keep the mistake, because it was too much work to change, but it also drew attention. Difference defies expectation. Difference draws attention.

Dad spent a lot of time at his garage. He and my mom fought constantly, usually about her long work hours and his unwilling-ness to help out around the house. Dad's interest in monogamy had been frail at best, and faded further with time and life and kids. Then my dad fell in love with the babysitter. She made the first move, according to him. The precipitating event for many life-changing decisions can often appear small, but triggers can be trivial when the conditions are just right. The babysitter's advance was all my father needed. Their relationship evolved quickly and passionately. It convinced him, he said, that if he could love some-one else so completely, then he must not love my mother any-more. "You can only love one person like that at a time," he said to me. Then, when the babysitter suddenly moved away less than a year later, Dad was devastated. He confessed everything to my mother and told her that he didn't love her anymore.

My mom wasn't about to let her marriage end without a fight. She'd witnessed her own parents' struggle and survival. Divorce wasn't supposed to be part of the plan. Dad didn't move out right away, but he did spend most of his nights away. For the next year he spent many of those nights at his favourite bar, before going back to his mother's house to sleep on the couch, late and drunk. Mom said that he never used to drink when he was happy, but Dad said that it helped him to be social. The truth was probably somewhere in the middle. Early on, nearly every night, he'd come home in time to tuck us into bed.

"Tuck, tuck, tuck," he'd say as he tucked the blankets tightly around me, securing me in comfort and warmth. Sometimes he'd just sit there next to me on the bottom bunk for a while. Then he'd go out into the kitchen and I'd fall asleep, listening to my parents scream at each other.

Sometimes there was no screaming. Sometimes he stayed the night, and it was almost like old times. On those beautiful, unpredictable mornings, Krista, Raymond and I woke up early and piled between him and Mom in their queen-size bed, and everything for a moment would seem normal again. We felt complete. On another of those unpredictable mornings, however, my mom had a seizure. She'd had them occasionally, especially when she was stressed or tired. Dad happened to be there that morning. He ran to the neighbour's house for help, Mom was taken to the hospital, and all of the tests came back inconclusive. She said she felt fine, and we didn't ask many questions. We were just grateful Dad was there.

That all ended for good when Dad met Joanne. Infidelity had become too powerful a habit. He got her pregnant and that made everything official. He moved his remaining things out of the house, and my first stepsister was born a few months later. It was generally understood that we weren't allowed to know her, even though we knew that she existed. We didn't see Dad much anymore either. It wasn't good or bad, it just was, a new normal, and we adapted. At least the fighting mostly stopped. We all missed my dad, my sister especially, but probably nobody missed him more than my mom. I had been conditioned to expect upset whenever he was around, because that's what usually followed his arrival at the house, so I didn't miss him as much.

For my fourth birthday party, my mother dressed me up in a crisp white shirt, black tie and bright-red vest. My sharp black dress pants were clean and pressed, at least at first. My then-fair hair was combed as evenly as possible, given the stubborn cowlicks at both the crown and the front of my hairline, a genetic force that seemed to afflict nearly all the Henick men.

We sat around the kitchen table, I and my family of aunts, and uncles, and cousins, and vaguely known though presumed relations, who usually came out to family events. A rectangular chocolate cake was set in front of me. It was slathered in brown frosting and piped unevenly around the edges with an unco-ordinated bright-blue icing. We had a few false starts to singing "Happy Birthday," thanks to a nearby cousin who was overeager to help me blow out my number four–shaped candle. I finally had her removed so that I could make my own wish.

My wish was the same short prayer I said every time we drove past Holy Redeemer, and every night before I went to sleep, and on every wishbone and shooting star I could find. I asked for my mom and dad to get back together. I blew out the candles, Mom snapped a picture, and she clicked the wheel on the camera that advanced the film forward. Another memory for the album she kept in her closet. She had one for each of us. My album was baby blue, she said, because I was her baby.

Still smiling for my mom with her camera in hand, I heard the familiar rumble of Dad's truck coming down Brooks Street. I felt a flutter in my stomach as I heard him turn the corner in front of our house on Lingan Road. I hurried to look out the big picture window behind me, just in time to see Dad's truck speed past. Joanne was in the passenger seat. His window was rolled down and his dark hair was messy in the wind. I remember his face, his smile, as he drove away. My shoulders fell and I felt a swell of hot tears in my eyes. I turned to my mother.

"Why didn't he stop?" I asked.

She paused for a moment, looking from the window back to me, her face an inscrutable mix of hurt and anger. Is she mad at me?

"I don't know, Mark," she said. "Maybe he was just in a hurry to get somewhere."

Later that night, as I was settling into bed, I could hear my mother talking on the phone in the kitchen, which was just on the other side of the wall from my pillow.

"How dare you drive by this house with that whore!" she screamed. "You couldn't even stop to say happy birthday?" She didn't wait for an answer. "I hope you're happy, you and that home wrecker!"

She slammed the receiver down. Then she picked it up again and slammed it back down two or three more times. I heard her crying through the wall. I probably would have gotten up to ask what was wrong, but Mom crying wasn't an unfamiliar sound anymore. I pictured her sitting on the kitchen floor, next to the side entrance, an image drawn more from memory than from imagination.

Soon the crying stopped. As quickly as it had started, it was over. I looked up to see my mother standing at my bedroom door. Mom was short, like the rest of the Costigans, and always complained about her weight. To me she was warm and comfortable. Her short, curly hair was a familiar silhouette in the hall light shining behind her. She'd taken off her glasses, and her pale-blue eyes looked tired and glossy, her cheeks pink, her small mouth forced into a thin smile that didn't match her expression.

I wanted to ask her what was wrong, but I didn't. Talking about our feelings wasn't against the rules; we just didn't do it.

My mom came over and sat on the side of my bed, careful not to bump her head on my brother's bunk above. Raymond went to bed later than me, so I rarely remember him being there.

"Did you have a good birthday, buddy?" Mom asked.

"Yeah," I said. I knew even then, in a childlike way, that was the answer she wanted and expected me to give. I didn't want to let her down. Life was hard enough without my complaints, but it also wasn't untrue. I didn't expect every part of everything to be perfectly good all the time—that would be no way to be happy. Childhood is like one long summer, even if it has a few cold days.

She paused for a long moment. "You know we'll always have each other, right?" she asked. "I'd do anything for you guys."

"I know, Mom," I said sleepily.

She sat silently for a minute longer. Then, reading my mind or knowing me well or falling back on habit, she lay down beside me. She pulled up the back of my pyjama shirt and ran her short nails across my back in the light, tickly way I liked. I closed my eyes and fell asleep.

My mother and father started divorce proceedings not long after. The divorce moved quickly. Unlike their marriage, there was relatively little fighting. Dad wanted a clean break, a fresh start. He told the court that he wanted nothing to do with any of us.

I didn't understand what we had all done wrong, and I can't remember anybody ever explaining it to me. When I overheard my mom talking to her close friend Helen about the annulment she was about to request from the Church—"Am I just supposed to pretend that the last fourteen years didn't happen?"—I remember thinking how that seemed like a lifetime. More than twice my lifetime, in fact. And since my mom had to ask the Church's permission to call off her marriage, I thought maybe they'd say no and everything would go back to the way it was. That's what I was praying for each time we drove by Holy Redeemer.

We were a working-class family at our best, but during and after the divorce and the annulment we were broke. Mom told us, a lot, that Dad never paid child support. She worked whatever extra hours she could get just to feed and clothe us, and we still needed welfare to survive. I didn't see it as easy or hard at the time; I was a little kid—it was just the way it was. We had beds to sleep in, toys to play with, and we were constantly surrounded by family. What did we have to complain about? The hard stuff? Well, everybody had it hard. This was Cape Breton. Sure, I missed my dad and wanted more of his attention, I didn't know why we weren't good enough for him to stay, and I didn't understand why even God couldn't seem to control the universe. But it could be worse.

We still went to church every Sunday, the front two pews of Costigans gradually expanding to the front four with the addition of another ever-growing generation. We still went to Nana Ag's house after mass, for homemade bread and her famous "magic soup." I'm not sure what made it magic—the memory maybe, the warmth. In the summer I played carefree with cousins in the backyard that bordered the steel plant, under the shadow of the overpass, where everything was painted some flaking shade of grey. I came in when called and sat in the chair where Papa Mike clutched his chest and died. I ate around the big chunks of tomatoes that Nana sometimes added to her soup. Tomatoes weren't part of the recipe; there was no recipe, she just happened to have tomatoes. She always caught me, and I always knew how she'd react.

"Look at 'im," she said. "Leavin' good soup behind!" You weren't expected to talk back to Nana Ag, ever, at all, so I stayed silent. She persisted. "What about them poor starvin' Biafrans?" she asked, almost certainly rhetorically. "They'd be glad to have a soup like that!"

I turned to my mother, sitting nearby. "Mom," I asked.

"Yes?" she answered, a thinly suppressed smile on her lips.

"What does 'Biafran' mean?" I was genuinely curious.

She looked at me for a moment, a faint, fond memory in her eyes. "It means eat your soup," she said.

Some battles were worth waging, but sometimes, Mom taught us, it was better just to eat your soup. We didn't have much, but it was everything we needed. We had each other. Wanting more at the risk of losing each other wasn't worth the fight. All of us grew from our roots, and those roots ran deep on Railroad Street.

My mom just wanted a normal life for her kids, even if life was hard, just like she'd had as a girl growing up in the duplex by the steel plant. She wanted to make a house a home, and to fill it with memories and hope and faith. She wanted peace.

Blessed are the peacemakers, said one of Nana Ag's little porcelain plaques.

For they will be called children of God.

CHAPTER 2

MY MOTHER WORKED A LOT OF EARLY DAYS AND late nights. She got up at five in the morning to be at the hospital for seven, usually leaving before I woke up. She often worked a twelve-hour day and got home by eight in the evening, just in time to see me off to bed. Whenever my mother worked a night shift, the pattern was reversed: she'd be gone at bedtime but home when I woke up. My mother was exhausted, stressed and sad all the time, but I hardly noticed—I was just a little kid. I liked the mornings after a night shift because she was home in time to have breakfast with us, and then she'd go to bed for the day while I was in school. When she had a string of days off, when she wasn't catching up on sleep, she spent her time catching up with us. I cherished those days, and quickly forgot about the others.

My sister, Krista, who was thirteen when Dad left, was the one who mostly cared for my brother and me in the gaps. Krista looked like my mother, soft and curly, but she acted more like my father—hard and blunt. She had a temper, she could talk a mile a minute, and she was never particularly interested in school. She was my best friend. When Krista became a teenager at the dawn of the nineties, she also became decidedly less enthusiastic about playing my mother.

Fortunately, it was also around that time that I started school. Finally having somewhere for me to go all day probably saved everyone a lot of trouble, not to mention money for babysitters. On my first day of primary—that's what we called kindergarten—my mother dropped me off at the first classroom on the left. Eastmount Elementary had only four classrooms, one each for primary through third grade. I entered the room and marvelled at the long green chalkboard and the big wooden teacher's desk. I turned and saw Mom still standing at the door. She had tears in her eyes. I waved goodbye, she waved back with her face drawn tight, and I made my way down the centre aisle. The room was a sea of little half-sized, one-piece wooden desks. I took my place at the one holding my name, written on a tent card, near the middle of the room.

The teacher, Mrs. O'Toole, had a reputation for being strict and cranky. I overheard some of the bigger kids calling her Mrs. Old Tool and I didn't think it was very nice. She always wore a button-down patterned dress and heavy glasses, and she seemed perpetually befuddled by the modern world. One time, in an exasperated fumble with a newfangled camera, she accidentally flashed a close-up picture of her own face. The class loved that and talked about it for days. I think she liked me; at least, that was still my default five-year-old assumption, that everyone liked me. She gave me very little evidence to support that assumption.

A few weeks in, I was colouring a picture of three ants crawling through blades of grass. We were learning about the colour black. I wasn't enjoying it, because black was my least favourite colour. I liked brighter, happier colours. I also couldn't focus because I had to go to the bathroom. I sat in my desk, trying my best to work, but the problem left unresolved only got worse. As the urgency inside me began to rise, my eyes darted around the room for options. They fell upon the clock near the door, which I still couldn't entirely understand. I got up and approached the front of the room, where Mrs. O'Toole was working at her big wooden desk.

"I have to pee," I said.

"Well, you'll have to wait," she replied, without looking up.

"But I really gotta go," I pled.

She glanced up at me over the big-framed glasses sliding down her nose. "The bell is going to ring in fifteen minutes," she said. "Go back to your desk and finish your work first."

I went back, picked up my black crayon and began scribbling all over the paper. Everything went black—the ants, the grass, the ground, the sky. I did what I was told. I brought the completed assignment back to the teacher.

"I'm done," I said. "Can I go to the bathroom now?"

Mrs. O'Toole looked at my work and was clearly not impressed. "For that, you can wait the ten minutes until the bell rings," she said sternly. "Go back to your desk."

I obeyed.

I felt a flush of panic wash over my face as I squirmed in my seat. I didn't know what else I could do. I had asked for help, but here I sat, helpless. About three minutes later, my bladder was at code-red, batten-down-the-hatches-level emergency of needing to pee. I was about to be embarrassed in front of everyone, I could see it coming, and I needed a plan to avoid that at all costs.

"Maybe I can just let a little out," I thought. This seemed a better alternative than literally exploding, right there in front of everyone, body parts everywhere. Just a little off the top, to buy me some time. Suddenly, I felt the warm stream down my leg. I willed every muscle in my skinny little body to turn it off, but it was stuck full open. There was no turning back. As urine started to pool on the floor, under the little basket of school supplies beneath my seat, the girl sitting in front of me looked back. Then she looked down. Then she quickly raised her hand.

"What is it, Nicole?" Mrs. O'Toole asked.

"Mark is peeing!" she shouted.

Everyone turned, stared at me, and laughed.

I sat there, frozen in place. Mrs. O'Toole glared at me from across the room, speechless, maybe in an attempt to scare my bladder into submission. It didn't work. The bell finally rang, and at last I felt relief. As kids got up and filed out to meet their parents waiting in the hall, I stayed in my seat, thoroughly shamed. The teacher came down the aisle and towered over me.

"Mark, what did you do?" she asked.

"I told you I had to pee," I answered matter-of-factly. *You Old Tool*, I added in my head.

It seemed like a dumb question. I asked for help, no help was given, so the problem got worse, and I peed my pants. It was a pretty elementary sequence of events.

With an exasperated huff, Mrs. O'Toole dismissed me. She escorted me and my wet pants to the hall, where my mother was the last parent waiting. The teacher explained what had happened, then turned and walked back into her room, toward the cupboard with the prearranged kit of rubber gloves, sawdust and disinfectant. I wasn't the first to do this, apparently. What was a horrible embarrassment for me was just another day on the job for Mrs. O'Toole.

I looked up at my mother. She looked down at me with a grin.

"I told her I had to pee," I said.

She nodded, we walked home together, and on the way she told me about the time an old nun did the same thing to her when she was my age.

She understood.

THERE WERE about four years each between my sister, my brother and me. However, because of the small schools in the Pier, we were never in the same one at the same time. This gave me space to find my own way, but there was also something comforting about having my siblings do things before me. Being able to watch my sister and brother attend a school before I did showed me it was safe. I was growing more reliant on predictability, more in need of safety and security. I didn't like feeling uncertain. I'd had enough uncertainty with Dad leaving and then, for a while, coming back unpredictably, and with Mom working shifts that some nights had her home for bedtime and some nights not.

Sometimes not being first to do something, or even second, gave me a sense of comfort but also the feeling I had something to prove. When I started first grade, as soon as Mrs. Jeans said I looked just like my brother and asked if I was as smart as him too, I felt a little more at ease. She wasn't a stranger anymore; she knew my brother. Even though we had just met, we were already bound by a shared connection. Thinking I had to prove that I was smarter than my brother gave me motivation, a goal toward which I could strive.

It'd been two years since Dad left. Mom worked a lot, and Krista was fed up with being our babysitter. She and Mom fought about it every day. My sister wanted to spend more time with her friends, especially her best friend, Carey. One weekend, Krista had planned to spend an entire day with Carey, but my mother told her that she needed to be home to watch us. My sister was furious. But Krista came home from school that day with a plan. After she and Carey had talked it over, she suggested to Mom that Carey's father, Gary, would be open to babysitting me and my brother. She didn't tell Mom that nobody had actually asked Gary.

Krista also didn't mention that Gary was newly single, though she and Carey talked about how much fun it would be if their parents got together. It would certainly solve a lot of problems, at least from Krista's point of view. Gary was about ten years older than my mother. He had worked most of his life in construction as a general labourer. It was manly work, and that suited him. He was strong and determined, with calloused hands and an unstoppable need to work, to build, to tear down, and to try again.

Gary Dalton's life had been shattered, however, the moment his skull was. One clear morning, he and his crew were putting the finishing touches on the roof of a new grocery store. He spotted a tool he needed a short distance away. He ran for it, but as he did, he passed over a sheet of plywood covering a still-unfinished section. The makeshift roof gave way beneath him and he fell through. He turned upside down in the air as he fell at least fifteen feet to the finished concrete floor below. He landed head-first. His skull, his face and pieces of tissue and brain exploded around him. He was rushed to the hospital, where he was wired, stapled and sewn back together.

Nobody expected him to live. Yet somehow, miraculously, bafflingly, he did. As his skull healed, there were noticeable peaks and valleys under his fair hair. There was an occasional hole, covered only by his weathered skin, especially at the front of his head where the initial impact occurred. He lost his senses of taste and smell as a result and was prone to violent migraines that would sometimes ravage him mercilessly for days on end. He took a variety of painkillers over the years, but they'd at best only take the edge off. Much of the damage was to his brain's frontal lobe, an area responsible for a wide variety of cognitive functions, including memory, personality, impulse control, social behaviours and mood regulation.

Shortly after his traumatic brain injury, while he was still recovering and around the time my dad left Mom, Gary's then wife, Jean, left him too. She took their five children and fled five thousand kilometres away. He said that he had no idea why they went. As he described the situation, it was completely unexpected that she could just run off with their family while he was practically on his deathbed. What was clear, however, was that Jean ran far, and she ran fast. Carey came back home to live with Gary about a year later, if it could still be considered her home after all that had changed. I imagine it was a hard transition for her too, not being around her mother or siblings anymore. Carey reconnected with Krista when she got back, and they quickly became close friends.

When Gary arrived one morning to drop Carey off at our house, he got hit with the preplanned request to babysit. Without hesitation, he agreed. That's the type of person he was, we learned: willing to help someone in need at a moment's notice. It was one of his many chivalrous traits. Then he agreed to help again, and many more times after that.

This was new for Mom, since Dad was never really one to help out like that. Gary's sense of responsibility filled a practical space in our lives, a structural void, a need for stability in changing waters. I think we served the same function for him. As Gary started coming around more, we began to depend on him more. Everyone wants to feel needed, some more than others. Mom needed someone to watch us, and he was reliable. It was mostly me and Raymond, since Krista was old enough to do her own thing. He made us chocolate cake, so he was fine by me.

About a year went by before my mother and Gary started dating. On their first date, he arrived in his big red pickup truck and drove her back to his place for a homemade dinner. He had mastered a few recipes during his recovery bachelorhood, including meat loaf and spaghetti and meatballs. His lemon meringue squares were perfect with the hot cup of tea that always came after a meal. Always orange pekoe, or "normal tea" as Mom called it, since that's what she knew. Not much in Cape Breton is fancy, first dates between middle-aged divorcees included.

When it was time to bring my mother home, Gary took a shortcut across Tank Road. It was an uninhabited, sparsely lit dirt road that cut past the big city water supply tank that gave the road its name. However, since it was little more than a service road, it was never well-maintained. For all the craters that dotted its surface, it was practically a route across the moon. One of Gary's more benign obsessive traits, it turned out, was avoiding every single pothole he encountered, even if he freely chose to drive on Tank Road, which presented him with hundreds of such encounters. It was a shortcut, after all.

Concentrating hard in the dark, he swerved wildly from one side of the road to the other. He drove along the gravel shoulder before jerking the wheel and sending the truck over to the wrong side of the road. When he came upon a particularly dense patch of potholes, he slowed the truck to a near crawl, easing the wheels down into each, then gradually climbing out again. On the other side of the hole he accelerated and resumed his swerving manoeuvres.

My mother, white-knuckled and clinging to her seat, didn't

say a word for the duration of the ride. When they arrived at our house, she said goodbye, got out of the truck and came inside. She didn't look back. The next morning, Mom gave Krista very specific instructions.

"If that maniac calls here again," she said, "tell him I'm dead."

But Gary was nothing if not persistent. After that date he started sending gifts, usually roses. He offered to babysit more regularly, and Mom usually agreed. She had someone who seemed to want her, and I can imagine how novel that felt. It didn't take long for him to wear her down. Maybe she was still on the rebound from her failed marriage. Maybe they both were. Someone who needs to feel wanted is a good match for some-one who wants to feel needed. As far as I was concerned, it was nice to have a more stable father figure around, like the ones my friends had, even if our own dad wasn't that far away. Everything seemed too good to be true.

Then, on one of the now-normal days that my brother and I were spending with Gary, he brought us along in his truck to visit a friend. From what I could gather, they had some work to do together. Gary received workers' compensation for the head injury that had left him unable to work in the eyes of the government, yet hardly a day went by where he wasn't working under the table for somebody. I don't think he knew how to not work. It was usually honest, hard, real man's work, as he described it: digging ditches, clearing trees, hauling loads of trash, or dirt, or snow, or whatever else needed moving, digging, cutting or building. That particular day he turned off the truck, got out and, through the open window, told us to wait where we were. His friend met him a few feet away.

As we sat in the driveway, I watched Gary—who was quickly starting to fill the void my father had left in our lives—talk to his friend. I listened to their conversation through the open truck window. I remember having a hard time reconciling what I saw with what I heard. What I saw was the nice man who had charmed his way into our lives with his old-world style. What I heard was a ranting tirade, peppered throughout with strings of expletives unlike anything I had ever heard before, even from Nana Marg, which was a high bar to meet. Someone had apparently done something of which Gary didn't approve, and his considerably less animated friend needed to hear him vent about it. It was probably how a "real man" really talked, but at that point it was completely incongruous with how I had come to know Gary. Two key factors in what controls attention are salience and relevance: is it obvious, and is it personally important? His behaviour was obvious because it was new, at least to me, and even that early on, Gary had become an important person in my life because of the need he filled.

I started to count each "fuck" that he said.

A few minutes later Gary returned to the truck, opened the driver's side door and hauled himself behind the wheel with a grunt. Even before he could shift the manual transmission into reverse, I voiced my observation in the amused tone of a kid who is fascinated by having heard something bad. "Did you know that you said the F-word twenty-six times when you were talking to that man?" I asked, with a mix of interest, surprise and mock scandal.

He stopped dead. He stared straight ahead, both hands on the steering wheel. After a long, silent moment, he turned toward us, his wide nose flared, chest rising and falling. The hardness of his face triggered an unexpected thump of my heart, and my breath caught in my throat. The situation suddenly wasn't just curious or funny anymore. My smile froze as he stared directly into my eyes. When he spoke, his voice seemed deeper than before.

"You better learn to mind your fucking business," he said.

I was seized with fear. It wasn't because of any obvious danger, necessarily, but rather due to the planted idea that there might be danger. That's one of my earliest memories of that feeling. Sure, I'd been afraid before—but not of someone with whom I assumed I'd be safe. My brother sat between Gary and me, in the middle seat of the red pickup's cab, and didn't say a word. He just looked out the front window, ignoring everything, or pretending to. Gary glared at me, unblinking, for a moment longer, the small muscles in his face saying far more than the big ones in his arms, shoulders and chest.

Then he turned and shifted the old truck into reverse. We backed out of the driveway and rounded the corner. Gary drove excruciatingly slowly down the bumpy dirt road that led us back to his house at the end of yet another long dirt road. We remained in silence for the entire ride. I was afraid to speak again.

Soon, though, Gary's kindness and usefulness in our lives made me forget all about the fear and shame he'd made me feel. Instead, I felt dumb and ungrateful for ever thinking ill of him. I doubted what I heard, regretted what I felt and eagerly forgave him. The last thing I wanted was for someone else to leave us, to leave me, especially someone so nice and helpful and stable.

For better or for worse, it was impossible not to like him.

NOTHING SEEMED certain in the years after my father left. Routine became my favourite armour against uncertainty. Routine was reliable, abundant and easy to invent. If I knew what was coming, then I would also know what, or who, wasn't.

I walked the same route to school every morning and the same way home every afternoon, day after day. From about five years old, rain or shine, I walked on my own down the same three-quarters of a kilometre on Lingan Road. There were never any concerns about safety. All the kids walked to school by themselves, and I made friends with a few of them along the way. I saw Andrew, Corey and Ian almost every day. They joined me in the morning and one by one took their leave on the way home. I knew when they were coming, I knew when they were leaving, and I knew when I would see them again.

Marilyn, the crossing guard, greeted me by name each morning when I crossed the three-way stop where Jamieson Street met Lingan Road. Whenever I found a lucky penny on the sidewalk, as I often did, I stopped at the little corner store to exchange it for a single one-cent candy. Cherry Blasters were my favourite. When I got to the playground, a few blocks farther, I cut through the still-shiny steel equipment to get to my school on the other side.

One morning, on another safe and familiar walk down this route that I knew so well, I didn't find a lucky penny, but I did find something new. I discovered my anxiety. I'm not sure how long it'd been waiting for me to find it. I'd had a dream the night before, so maybe I was primed to look for it anyway. In the dream, I found, hidden in a snowbank just before the playground by my school, a device that dispensed an unlimited supply of gold coins. I was so excited. When I woke up in the morning, I walked down Lingan Road to school and I searched everywhere for the gold. But it had been unusually warm and the snowbanks had all mostly melted. And of course it was only a dream. The distinction wasn't always clear to me. Still, I tried to dig in the icy remnants where I thought the dream gold had been. I gave up when I realized that the one chance I had to help my family was gone. I felt frustrated that I couldn't single-handedly finance our escape from all our troubles.

I crossed the playground and went to school. I felt tight inside. I was in second grade, and I had been struggling with cursive. We had a homework assignment due that morning, and the teacher would ask for it first thing. It was a simple sheet of drills, writing the letter *S* over and over again in cursive until it was seared into my muscle memory. Except that I hadn't done my homework. I hadn't done many of the other assignments before it either. I'd take them home, but if my mother wasn't there to help me, as she often wasn't, then they didn't get done. I had a small number of people with whom I felt safe, and for me safety had been conditioned to mean familiar. My familiar people didn't happen to have the skills or interest I needed. School wasn't Krista's thing. With Raymond, if I fell down, he was the one who tripped me rather than the person to help me up. I just assumed that's how big brothers were. Dad and Gary had both dropped out of school at a young age, so they couldn't do much for me either. I needed help, but in my immediate circle there wasn't a whole lot of help available, let alone offered.

The bell rang and, as feared, my teacher called for the homework first. I told her that I didn't have it. "Where is it?" she asked. "I don't know," I lied. I did know. It was in the trunk of Mom's Hyundai Pony, the one with the rust holes in the back floor through which we'd see the road speeding by. It was under the spare tire, with all the other incomplete assignments. I'd been stashing them there for weeks. It didn't seem irrational.

I felt embarrassed. I didn't want to let my teacher down again, and that's what I felt I was doing. I wanted to do the homework that was so important to her, something she reiterated each time I arrived to class without it. I wanted people to like me, teachers were important to me, and teachers liked smart kids who did their homework. The problem was, I didn't know how to do the homework, and I didn't have anyone whom I felt comfortable asking for help. My discomfort evolved into a fear of asking anybody for anything at all and then, gradually, just fear. Free-floating fear looking for a target toward which to direct itself.

Maybe I was overthinking it. I don't know why my mind started to work that way at such a young age, but it did. When I discovered anxiety—or when anxiety discovered me—I hated the uncertainty of not knowing how people might respond to me, to my weaknesses especially. What if my teacher won't help me? What if she hurts me instead, right when I need her most? What if she thinks I'm dumb? What if she doesn't like me? What if she too rejects me? My anxiety started with a persistent itch of *what-if*-ism.

I began struggling in other subjects. I dreaded bringing home quizzes and assignments for the requisite parent signature because I didn't want my mother to see that I was struggling. Each day, I came back from school filled with fear. We didn't talk about how we were doing at school; it wasn't disallowed, it just wasn't normal. Besides, she had so much to worry about as it was, I didn't want her to worry about me too. I was fine. Mom was at work most days when I got home from school anyway, so I was able to avoid the problem for a long time.

Fortunately, I had my big sister to look out for me. She wasn't the type to hold my school difficulties against me. If anything, my problems bonded us more. Krista neatly etched perfect reproductions of our mother's signature on the top of my most recently failed tests. *Brenda Costigan-Henick*. Mom had reintroduced her maiden name to her signature but did so gradually. "I don't want to have a different name than my kids," she said to her friend Helen one Saturday at our kitchen table. She practised her newly hyphenated signature a few times on a piece of scrap paper in blue pen, in her perfectly even Catholic school–drilled cursive.

That change to my mother's name made me very uncomfortable. I didn't want to see her new name on the top of my failed assignments. I didn't want her to know I was having a hard time at school. I didn't want to be held back, or to be left behind.

I didn't want any more change.

CHAPTER 3

MOM AND GARY SUDDENLY DECIDED TO LIVE TOGETHER. At least, it seemed sudden to me, because I didn't see it coming. One night I was sleeping in my own bed, the next night I was sleeping in a strange new place.

I don't remember anyone explaining to me what was happening, or why. I don't think my parents' divorce was even finalized yet. But when Gary decided he had a job to do, we saw that he preferred to get it done fast. The move itself happened so quickly—a whole house in a single school day, it seemed—that I don't really remember moving at all. Krista came home one day to find all our things in the back of Gary's red pickup truck, on the way over to his house.

It felt as though we were expected to see the move as a great thing. Not that long ago we were struggling to afford food and bills, but now—thanks to Gary —we could have a more normal life. Except that this was an entirely new normal. My routines, which kept my anxiety and insecurity and uncertainty at least partly at bay, were suddenly gone. Still, even if my input was neither requested nor required, part of me was open to the adventure of our new life. It was a chance to start over.

Gary lived in a square, yellow-and-brown, two-storey home, the last house at the end of a dead-end dirt road. The house was surrounded on three sides by more than a hundred acres of his mostly empty property. Other than the house, there was a kilometre-long gravel driveway with a shipping container–sized tool shed about halfway down, and some old cars and other discarded equipment where the driveway curved to an end at a clearing in the trees. The stuff that went down there was the stuff Gary didn't want anyone who happened to visit or drive by to see. The rest of the property was rolling, immaculately groomed grass fields, which gave way to thick coniferous forest as far as the eye could see.

Gary tended to his land obsessively. Over the years, he had added adjacent plots as they became available. His house was on the original plot where he had grown up, which he had inherited from his father. His childhood house had long since been torn down to build this one, where he had raised his first family. The fourth side of his property, facing the only neighbour and the only way back up the dirt road, was bordered by a long wooden rail fence. The other side was the neighbour's horse corral, and his little blue house beyond that. Gary's brother lived there, but we didn't talk about him.

My previous home on the corner of Lingan and Brooks wasn't in a particularly busy area, but at least it was inhabited. We had immediate neighbours nearby in every direction. There was only one big pine tree in the front yard, one that Mom and Dad had planted together when they first moved there. At Gary's place, there were so many trees that they all blended together into one big mass of forest. There were no cars or sirens speeding by on the dead-end road. There was definitely no rumble of my father's truck coming around the corner.

For the most part, there was only silence at Gary's house. At night, there was near-total darkness. Two fat concrete cylindrical light poles oriented the opening of the driveway, and two skinnier ones helped to locate the long walkway to the side door about a hundred feet in. The first twilight at what was to be my new home, I sat out in the grass and listened to a loon call carrying over the trees and hills all the way from Brown's Lake. Sometimes when I went out there, I could hear the *pop pop pop* of rifles at the shooting range, somewhere on the other side of the forest. A lot of the time I heard only the overwhelming screams of peeper frogs from every direction. After nightfall, once the screaming mostly stopped, the only thing I heard was my own heartbeat, the only thing I saw were the stars. It was easy to let my imagination carry me someplace else.

I went inside to my strange new bedroom. We had visited Gary's house lots of times over the last few months, so the basement where my room was located wasn't unfamiliar. I just hadn't realized how low and damp and cold it was. Even though the bed had my Ninja Turtle sheets, it wasn't my mattress in my bunk bed where I lined up my stuffed animals for the recurring wedding of Brownie Bear to Pinky Rabbit. Pinky was still my favourite comfort, and we were practically inseparable, especially at night. At night here, the walls made noises, different noises, not the ones I was used to. The pipes and wood groaned and creaked, tapped and clunked. The sound of footsteps carried through the ceiling, and I couldn't tell right away whom they belonged to or picture in my mind what they must be doing.

Most of our belongings were stored down in the tool shed. Pinky Rabbit was put there, with the rest of what Gary called our "junk." My brother later told me that Gary had burned it all, the stuffed rabbit included, in one of the big garbage fires he had in the clearing around the bend. It wasn't unusual for Raymond to say things like that to me, true or not. Yet whatever he told me always seemed entirely rational to me at the time.

"You're too old to be playing with stuffed animals," Gary responded when I asked where Pinky had gone. "Besides, it was pink. Pink is for girls," he said. "And faggots."

He didn't say unkind words unkindly, but I felt shame anyway. It was my fault for asking, for being weak. "Be a man," Gary told me, especially if he sensed I might cry. From as early as second grade it was a refrain he repeated to me often. *Be a man.* The words took root and quickly grew into a permanent echo in my head, first in his voice and then, gradually, in my own. Whenever I showed him that I could suck up whatever was bothering me, I earned a rewarding look of approval from him. At seven years old, I learned to crave his highest praise: that I was "a real little man."

I didn't want to lose that honour, so I learned not to talk about how I was really feeling, to hardly even show it, especially if I was feeling sad. I'd been increasingly anxious about asking for help even before the routines and things that gave me comfort were taken away. Now I couldn't even say or show how I was feeling. When typical, otherwise unremarkable challenges came up—and they always came up, life is hard after all—I looked around for options to address them, but I often found none. Upsets and strong emotions started to feel as though I was bursting into flames in a locked room full of empty fire extinguishers.

So, out of necessity, I happened upon a way to cope that nobody could take away from me. I became more introverted and closer to my thoughts. In my imagination I could escape or entertain myself however I wanted, without fear or judgment or shame or loss. I could do it in secret, just slip away for a while, and no one would be the wiser. My inner life was mine, to create as I dreamed, and nobody else could judge it, or change it, or take it away from me. I was in complete control of the world I was building inside me—at least at first.

School hadn't taken summer break yet, so I was bused, or driven, from Gary's to Eastmount for the final few weeks of class. I was still struggling with cursive, and I had gotten so far behind on the take-home assignments that my teacher disciplined me regularly for it. I didn't mind staying in at recess. I didn't know how to catch up or fix my homework problem when I was in so deep anyway. I was stuck, and there wasn't much else I could do.

Our little Hyundai Pony with the fire-engine-red paint job was parked at the very end of the long driveway, as far away from the house as possible. As I was getting to know my new home and exploring the vast, empty wilderness that surrounded it, my adventures increasingly took me down there. Every time I went down and caught sight of the old car, I felt a hot flash of shame and guilt about the collection of unfinished assignments hidden away under the spare tire in the trunk. The thought of them throbbed in my head like a telltale heart. But I ignored the feeling and, instead, explored the forest line at the end of the driveway. Gary seemed to be able to escape into nature, so maybe I could too. Eventually, I started to wander beyond the driveway down the grassy path that Gary had cleared between the trees, before retreating back to the house.

By the time I finished second grade, I was glad finally to be free of the secret hidden assignments. My brother and I had a tradition on grading day at the end of each school year. After we received our report cards, we went up to my father's garage at Nana Marg's house. In the yard, between the dozens of scrapped or nearly junked cars—Dad didn't enjoy the effort involved in painting anymore and resorted mostly to scrapping cars for parts instead—my father had cut an old barrel in half lengthwise and set it up on its side.

We loaded our most recent school year's worth of old homework, assignments and sometimes even a few books into the barrel, poured gasoline over it all, then set it on fire. The fire was purifying. It was a chance to start afresh. Dad was still a big advocate for fresh starts, and the ritual allowed us to start our summers as carefree kids. That first summer living with Gary, I went down to the old Pony at the end of his driveway, dug out the cursive assignments and slipped them into my pile for the fire. I burned my shame.

In summers past, I'd spent my time running around with my friends, having sleepovers and taking trips to our musty bungalow in Big Pond. The windowsills there were lined with hundreds of dead houseflies and the beach was too rocky and tangled with seaweed to swim, but it was always nice to get away. The bungalow was gone now. The last time I had stood in the kitchen there, I watched my mom and her friend Helen, sitting at the table, writing *FOR SALE* on a blank piece of lined yellow legal pad with a big red marker. My mother stuck it to the front door as we were leaving, probably more for my father to find than to attract any buyers. As we drove away, I heard her laugh, even though nothing seemed all that funny.

I didn't keep in touch with any of my friends that summer, even my best friends, since I hadn't been able to walk to school with them for a while. It was a small change in my routine, but small changes reverberate and accumulate. I was isolated in the woods now and couldn't easily walk to my friends' houses. When people and places and things weren't easily accessible, they might as well not have existed at all. Like my cursive homework, or my dad. Out of sight, out of mind.

Without much else to do, I had a lot of time to myself to spend with my memories and ruminations. Being alone and feeling alone are kind of a chicken-and-egg thing, and in the earliest days of depression it's hard to tell which is which. That's one reason I didn't realize I was becoming depressed. Then again, I wouldn't have known what to look for or what to call it if I had noticed. I was too young to know what many of my emotions and experiences were called. Gary's house was, at times, the perfect place to feel lonely, especially when his kids were back in town.

Although his ex-wife had fled to Alberta with the kids, it didn't take long for them to start coming back. They didn't usually stay longer than a few weeks or months at a time before leaving again. I never thought much about why they came and went from their perspective; I was too caught up in my own life. I guess we had a little more in common than I realized. Each of them in turn, sometimes overlapping, returned to the house for periods of time: Gary's eldest, Dwayne, and Little Gary—who was hardly little, he was an accomplished bodybuilder—along with Gary's daughters, Lorraine and Carey, and his youngest son, Matthew, who was only about a year older than me.

I sensed Gary's preference for his first family, and I'm certain that Krista, Raymond and even my mom did too. He didn't exactly try to hide it. Whenever the prodigal children returned, we were reminded that we were the visitors, not them. We were the substitute family. Whenever one of Gary's kids wanted something that we had, his decision—or his unrelenting pressure on Mom to make the decision—always favoured his kids over us.

Contrary to the gregarious, engaging, storytelling character that Gary portrayed to everyone beyond the dead-end dirt road, the man I noticed after we moved in didn't seem to be an especially social person. He seemed most content when he was alone, picking rocks from his field and clearing brush from his forest. He behaved differently, I thought, when people were watching. I did too. I can't speak for Gary, but in my case there was a growing disparity between the life I lived in front of others and the one I lived inside myself. More and more, I preferred the life inside my head.

I never fully let go of my prayer for everything to go back to normal, even if that so-called normal had only ever been all in my head.

ONE EVENING, Mom was watching television in the den, as she and Gary did most evenings. They usually watched *Wheel of Fortune*, though reruns of *All in the Family* or *Three's Company* weren't uncommon. The lights were all off, and only the glow of the TV lit my mother's face as she sat on the couch across from it. Gary emerged from their bedroom and went into the kitchen.

He called Raymond and me upstairs to join him, then he knelt down to talk to us. It was probably the first and only time he ever did that, but I think it was less a consultation and more to let someone in on the surprise he'd planned. From the pocket of his best pair of work-worn jeans he produced a dainty little black velvet box. He opened it and showed us the engagement ring that he was about to offer our mother. It had one big diamond in the middle, flanked by a smaller one on either side, set into a white gold band.

We knew what it meant. I was overjoyed. Finally, I thought, we would have a father again. That, surely, would make everything feel normal. We'd get to be part of the first family. Gary told us to wait while he went into the den and closed the door. Through the yellow-frosted glass panels in the door I saw the glow of the television go dark. I heard the muffled voice of Gary asking my mother to marry him.

"I guess so," she answered.

Gary opened the door, smiling. I ran to him, laughing, cheering and tugging at his arm.

Mom looked shaken. I hugged her. I was so happy and couldn't contain my giddiness.

"Way to go, DAD!" I said, jumping up and down.

It was the first and last time I ever called Gary that.

I STARTED third grade at South Bar Elementary.

It was closer to Gary's house than Eastmount had been, but it was in a small bedroom community in the opposite direction. Sometimes Gary's mail came addressed to Sydney, sometimes South Bar, because we were somewhere between the two.

South Bar was nestled along a highway on the edge of a cliff that looked out toward where Sydney Harbour opened onto the Atlantic Ocean. Depending on the tide, sometimes you could see the raised ridge of the sandbar that jutted up from the ocean floor and gave the community its name. Little Gary took us to the beach nearby a few times that summer, if you could call it a beach. It was an outcrop of the cliff where, on a calm day, the lapping water's edge revealed an underlying bed of jagged rocks and the occasional shard of blunted sea glass. Farther out, purple jellyfish bobbed up and down on the high swells of the bracing cold salt water. We'd heard that a few people had died, or at least had heart attacks, plunging into that water. On the side of a steep hill, before the cliff, was South Bar Elementary.

My new school felt a lot bigger because it went all the way up to grade six, not just to grade three like Eastmount. There was a gym, a library and even a computer lab. None of my family had gone to school there, and nobody knew me, so I felt like more of an outsider than I had expected on the first day. In my first few weeks, I got back a multiplication test with a big zero marked in red pen at the top. I wasn't ready for my new school or my new grade. I cried in the middle of class. My teacher and some of the other kids tried their best to comfort me.

"It's okay, Mark," the teacher said. "You just need a little extra time and help to catch up."

It felt nice to be comforted. I wasn't used to encouragement. I didn't know how to respond to it. Nobody there seemed to expect me to be a man or to suck it up, and that was good because expectations were important to me, both assuming them and meeting them. I was able to express my emotions without being reprimanded. It was only a simple moment, a small, tender connection, but it went a long way toward making me feel welcome in a strange new environment.

Those moments of comfort and connection remained less common at Gary's house, and it took a lot longer for me to settle in to our still-new arrangement there. Even though we had met Gary through him babysitting me and my brother, I'm not sure he fully appreciated the fact that Mom's kids were part of the package when we moved in and he proposed. Now he was outnumbered, and by Henicks at that. That's what seemed to bother him the most. We heard a lot about "The Henicks" from him, even from the earliest days.

"Marg Henick is a direct descendant of Hitler," Gary said. "Henicks are Nazis." He said it to me with a big, unhappy-looking smile one evening while Mom was at work. He always said stuff like that with a smile, and his smile made me feel bad for feeling bad. The few times I did say that something bothered me, or if I told Mom about it, he had built in enough plausible deniability to have his behaviour dismissed as innocent teasing. He'd follow up by doing something nice or giving me something, so that I almost felt rewarded for feeling bad. "Be a man," he'd say. "Learn to take a joke." Then he'd do it again and the cycle repeated.

Gary "joked" about the Nazi thing a lot. He said it often enough that I believed him. In third grade we had an in-class assignment to design a family crest. On mine I drew a swastika, having no idea what it really meant. My teacher saw it as he walked by, and he knelt down at my desk. He inspected my drawing closely, then looked at me.

"Mark, you can't put that on there," he said gently.

"Why?" I asked.

"Because the Nazis were very bad people," the teacher answered.

It suddenly all made sense to me. If Nazis were very bad people, I thought, and Henicks were Nazis, then Henicks were very bad people. "I'm a Henick, so that must mean I'm a very bad person." Gary was a convincing storyteller, and I internalized a lot of the stories he told. I internalized almost everything.

In our family, I was the sensitive one. Krista was the feisty one and Raymond was the smart one. Mom was proud of each of us for our unique gifts and never hesitated to tell anyone who would listen. I was "the baby" to my mother's friends. They all said that Krista would pick a fight with the devil himself, while Raymond was a genius, gifted at math especially, but also a talented artist.

Mom was generally blind to our shortcomings. Krista's attitude and propensity for backtalk often got her into things over her head. Raymond was the middle child and could be calculating and resentful of people who he thought had received benefits that he hadn't. Krista wasn't the type to put up with Raymond's shit—or anyone else's for that matter—so he mostly took his frustrations out on me. I was needy and craved reassurance, and without it I was becoming increasingly introverted, afraid and insecure.

We'd been living at Gary's place for about three years, and I shared my little bedroom in the basement with my brother. His single bed was on one side of the room, mine on the other, and between them there was a second door to the bedroom that my sister shared with Carey. They had to walk through our bedroom to get to theirs. I didn't mind sleeping in my sister's lobby; I liked having her close because it made all the noises at night seem less scary. I wanted to be close to my brother too, but he never seemed to share those feelings.

I was in fourth grade at South Bar, and otherwise settled, with the exception of having acquired my first bully. It started when the fat little red-headed kid got me on the ground and sat on my back, making it impossible for me to breathe. In the winter he grabbed me by the hair and hit my head on the ice. The grounds supervisor sometimes came to help, but it was always too late. I probably put up with it for so long because the kid was my friend. He was quiet, awkward and an outcast like me. I didn't want to lose any friends, so I didn't say anything. I was a lot like my mom that way. *Blessed are the peacemakers.*

The school bully didn't really bother me that much. I had ways of avoiding him if I needed to, and I had safe people around me, teachers and staff whom I liked and trusted. He wasn't my only friend, either. I had made some others, though I rarely went to any of their houses after school or invited them to mine. What bothered me more were the bullies at home, especially Gary, and to a lesser extent my brother. I couldn't avoid them as easily.

Things really started to unravel with my brother first.

He was never especially nice to me and at best ignored me completely, but then he started to become more aggressive. Raymond's aggression toward me was only occasionally physical. He wasn't very physically imposing and I think that, with Gary's help, Raymond was self-conscious about that. Instead, his tactics were more often psychological. Raymond was smart. If he wanted me to do something, he just threatened to tell Mom about some bad thing that I had done, some lie I'd told, some secret I held. He knew most of these details because I'd told him. He was my big brother and I trusted him.

I had a desperate need for connection at all costs. I possessed an eager willingness to prioritize validation and acceptance over just about anything. I wanted to be seen, to feel seen. I wanted most what I was given the least, which I think made it easier to take advantage of me. That may have been at least part of the reason why Raymond was able to exert such powerful control over me when he found out I'd been molested by a boy a few years older than me. As I got a little older myself, it compounded inside me, and it became my dirtiest, most shameful secret. I didn't realize until much later how I had internalized this shame and how profoundly something I hid from almost everybody else had deeply affected me. I tried to pretend it wasn't a big deal, but for me, it was.

The molester was the son of a family friend, and the incidents happened during a series of sleepovers at his house. I was about seven years old when the first incident took place, and it was repeated several times over the following two years or so. I didn't understand what was going on during these episodes. I visited

their house many times, sometimes with my whole family, sometimes alone, but not often since it was a long drive away. Gary
came with us on one of the overnight trips not long after he and
Mom started dating. It was well-known by everyone that Gary
couldn't sleep in any bed but his own. So he got up and left in the
middle of the night and drove home, leaving us stranded there.

My friend was a few years older than me. On one of the trips,
we lay together in his top bunk, in the room he shared with his
younger brother. When he kissed my face, sloppily, he told me it
was a game, that we were pretending to be puppies. He kissed my
neck and my chest and licked his tongue over my body. Then he
rubbed his hands all over me, and slid them up my shirt. He never
tried to take my pants off; that came later, when someone else did
it to me again, one of my ninety-four or so cousins.

I went along with it. It felt weird and sticky and kind of gross,
but I didn't know that I was supposed to say no. I didn't know that
I could. It was an unusual game, one I'd never played before, and I
was curious. One of the times we were playing, his mother opened
the bedroom door and he jumped up quickly. "Lunch is ready," his
mother said. She didn't notice, or pretended not to. We got down
from the bed and ate grilled cheese sandwiches and tomato soup,
and everything went on as normal. After a while it started to feel
shameful and wrong, in no small part because of Gary's frequent
admonitions against same-sex relations as evil. But I felt it had
been going on for too long by then for me to say anything.

Besides, whom would I tell? I was constantly surrounded by
Gary's rigorously enforced culture of hyper-masculinity and a
peculiar religiosity. The sermons that set the tone of his culture
were frequently delivered to us from his pulpit at the head of the
kitchen table. They were laced with a strict, seemingly subjective morality. He preached devotion to the Church, and he was

confounded by homosexuality. "Man shall not lie with another man! That's in the Bible!" How could I possibly tell him that I'd been molested by a boy? He'd already taken to calling me a "fag" because of my perceived weakness. If I told him that boys seemed to pay more attention to me than girls, and that I didn't entirely know how I felt about that, I was afraid he'd kill me.

Yet, for all his preaching and ostentatious religious statuary, I remember Gary taking us to mass only once. My brother and I were horsing around, it embarrassed him, and he never went back. I guess we had shattered the illusion of perfection that he seemed to seek. We never pointed out that he didn't go to mass; in fact, as an altar boy, I myself went far more. It wouldn't have mattered anyway. Gary's sermons didn't even have to make sense. There wasn't usually any time for a question-and-answer session; these were not discussions. Gary needed to vent, and we needed to listen. Maybe it made him feel less alone on his journey, to take captives along the way.

One day, in the den between the Resurrection painting and the statue of the big, bloody body of Christ, Raymond and I were arguing about something long since forgotten. My mother was listening nearby. Raymond had found out about what I had come to consider the dirty and shameful game I had played with my friend. When he did, rather than step in, stand up for me and put an end to it, he used it against me. It had become one of his most reliable tools of extortion. Whenever he wanted me to obey, the mere mention of "the Game" brought me into line. The argument this day, however, must have been important enough to me that I either stood my ground more firmly than usual or felt safer to do so with Mom there. My brother didn't like to be challenged. In a momentary lapse of reason, Raymond finally overplayed his hand.

"The Game . . ." he sneered, his eyes a hateful squint filled with triumphant expectation.

"What's the Game?" Mom interjected, looking from my brother to me.

My eyes widened and I felt a lump catch in my throat. Raymond smiled, almost certainly thinking he had won. Something inside me overflowed. I just couldn't hold it in.

"Tell her!" I screamed. "I don't care, tell her!"

Raymond's expression turned panicked and petty. "Fine, I will," he said, but his voice had lost the confidence it had before. Mom still looked confused. With a frustrated, cathartic huff, I turned on my heel and stormed outside.

I stalked down the walkway, down the driveway, past the midpoint shed. I went down around the bend by the old red Pony, down the grassy path and into the woods. I followed the path until I came to the thick, full wall of trees at the end. Then I stopped. I heard birdsong in the branches and a trickle in the distance. The early summer sun cast down shadows through the leafy canopy overhead. I hated feeling so much, too much. It was cooler down here.

I didn't want anyone to find out about this shameful thing I had been part of. I felt trapped and afraid, but I knew I couldn't ask for help. If I did, I might regret it. The people whom I loved might think differently of me, they might leave me, and I couldn't risk any change to the few close connections I had.

I don't know what Raymond did after I left, if he told my mother my dirty, sinful secret. Nobody talked to me about it later. But two things did happen: my brother stopped using the Game to control me, and I never again went to my friend's house by myself.

Speaking up apparently changed something, even if I didn't realize it at the time.

CHAPTER 4

WITH SEPTEMBER COMING, I WAS GETTING READY TO start fifth grade at South Bar. That meant I was almost one of the big kids, near the top of the food chain in the elementary kingdom. That position came with a certain status and responsibility, and I liked that idea. My mother was going to take me out to get new school supplies in the morning. However, I knew it wasn't going to happen this particular August morning as soon as I heard Gary and my mom arguing when I came up the stairs from my room in the basement.

"Why don't you just call up Jean, since you still love her so much," Mom yelled. "Have her come back, and you can be happy, and everything can go back to normal." She always cried when she screamed.

"You don't think she would?" Gary shouted back. His voice was spiteful, mocking.

Gary rarely talked about his life before his ex-wife, Jean. It seemed as if that's where his life stopped, stayed stuck in suspended animation. While in the sermons he'd repeat the same few stories about his youth and childhood before his marriage, the rest was left largely blank. Maybe nothing interesting happened. But what I started to learn is that everybody has different ways of coping with a past they'd rather forget. The only possible history that we had heard on this—from Nana Marg, of course, whom we all knew as the Queen of Rumour—was that Gary's father used to hang around at the Henick house on Blueberry Hill with her husband, my grandfather. I'm not sure if the moonshine tunnels under the house were still running then, but Gary's dad apparently used to go over whenever they got to drinking in the kitchen, according to Nana Marg, which was a lot. That said, Nana Marg also had a joyful habit of sowing discord, perhaps as a remnant of her own less than predictable life.

Mom and Gary's fights often seemed to come out of nowhere. The trigger would be so meaningless that I wouldn't even see the fight coming. I thought it was my fault for not paying attention. To me, some days, Gary just woke up wrong and I knew by his silence or his tight, fast body movements that it was going to be a dark day. Those days seemed to coincide with his head-trauma-related migraines. Occasionally there was more of an aura leading up to one of his migraines or moods, whichever came first. It was a change in the way he told jokes or the content of his stories, warnings like the first leaves that fall as the days turn darker and colder. Gary was often friendly and assertive, outgoing and funny. But when the dark days came, with or without warning, they were frequent and unpredictable and intense enough to require at least some level of constant self-defensive vigilance. I wasn't always sure which Gary I'd be dealing with on any given day.

Mom and Gary's fights didn't always even start as fights. More often, they began with Gary rigidly fixating on and obsessively pushing some trivial thing. At least, it seemed trivial to me. In those moments, whatever the target issue, it was obviously important enough to him to be worth creating so much tension. The triggers often related to some way that things were supposed to be, according to Gary, rather than how they actually were or were becoming.

Mom had been trying to nest ever since we moved in, to make Gary's house feel more like our home too. She wanted the place to have a little more warmth, to be closer to what she was comfortable calling a home. She started by moving some furniture around and adding a few decorations that she liked, but when Gary came home, the furniture was always moved back and the decorations were taken down. So my mother started making smaller changes instead—the silverware in the drawer, or which throw pillows were on the couch. But Gary's attention to detail was exacting, as though his loss of taste and smell had heightened his sense for change. He was always in complete control of our environment. This was especially true for the red-carpeted living room between their bedroom and the kitchen. Mom used to call it Gary's Shrine of St. Jean. Whatever she changed would be back to the "right" way within hours.

We all assumed, and he never denied it, that the right way was his ex-wife's way. It seemed that our family's only function was to re-create Gary's pre–head injury life. I think it bothered him that Mom had still been using the Henick name, albeit hyphenated. It might have looked to the outside world as though she were one of The Henicks, and how the outside world saw us seemed to be very important to him.

As far as we could tell, Mom still wasn't ready to have a different name from her kids, because her kids were the most important thing to her, as she told us all the time. When Mom made her own decisions like that, it also made it harder to turn her into "Jean Two," as she sometimes called herself to people like her friend Helen, who was in on the joke. Krista used to tease my mother that she shouldn't be surprised if she woke up some morning to find that Gary had styled her hair in her sleep to make her look more like his ex-wife. That became a running joke too, and it felt good to laugh about it because it was the only way we could talk about it. The laughter was cathartic.

It wasn't just Mom, or the house, but rather the whole world that needed to conform to Gary's expectations. His need for control was a constant source of friction between him and my mother. In fact, they probably ended up arguing more regularly than my mother and father ever did. If my father had not impregnated another woman and moved out, there would have been time for them to make up the gap. I still would have preferred it that way, and continued to pray for them to get back together, even if not every day anymore. Whenever Mom and Gary argued, Mom always gave in, against her wishes and better judgment, to avoid prolonging the fight. She always wanted to keep the peace. "That's just the way he is," she'd say.

It was clear to us that Gary would do just about anything to make our image fit his narrative of the happy little family in the country, with a big strong provider man and a good little woman by his side. Those were the general themes of his favourite country songs and western movies. Except, as we eventually learned, Gary had fought with his first family too. We had heard about how Jean had left him frail and on the verge of death, and that she detonated their allegedly perfect little life without warning. But hints gradually emerged that their perfect little life hadn't been so perfect after all.

By the time I started grade five in September, things around the house were tense, especially between Gary and Raymond. Gary got agitated when my brother's showers ran too long—

which was anything over ten minutes. When that happened, he would stomp down to the basement, go into the furnace room under the stairs and shut off the main valve for the hot water while Ray was in the shower. This happened a few times a week. Whenever he could, Ray would shower when Gary wasn't home. Each of us tried to find our own ways to adapt and cope, for as long as we could.

Patience, however, was notoriously not one of Raymond's strengths, and he was the first to leave. The last straw came one evening while Mom and Gary were out for dinner. Krista and Carey were watching a movie in the den, and Raymond was upstairs with them. At some point Ray offered to make the girls a pizza, which they could all eat with the movie. It had become a routine for us, whenever we were having a movie night, to enjoy homemade pizza along with it.

Raymond assembled the ingredients. Making a pizza isn't complicated, and he enjoyed it and was good at it. But he seemed to like the opportunity to be useful even more. When he was done, he served up the pizza, ate, then went to bed for the night. It had been, up to that point, an uneventful evening. Gary and Mom arrived back home a little over an hour later. They were hardly through the door when it became clear what kind of mood Gary was in.

"Who was cooking?" he asked. He used his loud, authoritarian, electrically charged voice whenever a storm was coming. Although he couldn't smell or taste as a result of the brain damage, Gary had told us how he could "sense" changes in the air and "feel" certain spices in his mouth.

"Who was cooking?" he asked more loudly, his chin tilted up to get a better sense.

He slipped off his shoes at the mat; he couldn't violate his own strict rules about no shoes in the house, unless, of course, he was in a better mood or it was a visitor from the outside who didn't live there. He came into the kitchen from the porch and passed the open door where Krista and Carey were still watching television. That's when he saw the dirty pizza pan in the sink. We didn't know why—triggers are sometimes trivial—but the sight of the pan ignited him.

"Who made pizza?" Gary demanded, clearly enraged.

"Ray did," Carey answered.

"He made it for us," Krista added, but it was too late.

Gary turned fast and barrelled past them, out of the kitchen and down the stairs. He turned left at the first door in the basement and barged into the room that I shared with my brother. Raymond had heard Gary's booming voice at the top of the stairs and ran to his bed and hid under the blankets. He had history with Gary's temper and he knew enough to be afraid. Gary pulled back the sheets and grabbed him with both hands by the shirt. He yanked him up and out of the bed easily—Gary was still strong. He dragged my brother by his shirt, backwards up the stairs. Ray was still half-asleep, but when Gary slammed him against the wall, he was instantly awake, terrified and confused.

My brother kicked and wriggled, but it was no use, Gary's hands were like a vise. His nine calloused, meaty fingers were tangled up in the shoulders of Ray's shirt. Gary had been around fourteen when he lost the finger. He and some friends were racing down a steep hill on a homemade go-kart—really just a slab of heavy metal with poorly attached wheels, no steering, no brakes. As it accelerated, his fingers curled around the steel front edge to get a better grip. When the front wheels came off, the front of the go-kart came crashing down on the ground, grinding off a few fingers as it continued down the hill. Gary was embarrassed to admit to his own father what had happened, lest he think he was weak. By the time he got to the hospital, the doctor was able to reattach only two of the three detached or dangling fingers. The third was ground down to the knuckle.

Now he had my brother pinned against the wall. Gary's eyes went glassy when he got into a state like this, as if he was a different person. His lips were wet, and white spittle accumulated in the corners of his mouth. His lips twisted up into a snarl, his teeth bared. His anger was never manic or scattered; it was directional, powerful and intentional. He was an unstoppable charging bull when someone had, unknowingly, waved a red flag in his mind.

Mom was screaming for him to let Raymond go. He relented, just for a moment. Mom's voice could still do that. A moment was all Raymond needed to break free. He jerked away, bolting past Mom, out the door, and fled into the night, up the dirt road, with nothing but socks on his feet. Mom chased after him, but it was no use, he wasn't coming back. Ray slept at a friend's house that night.

The next day, about mid-morning, Mom brought me along for the drive to the house where my brother had fled. She parked the car in the sloped gravel driveway outside the big white house in Sydney River. There was a tall set of faded wooden stairs on the side of the house, leading up to the grey aluminum door. "Stay here," she instructed.

I obeyed. When she was terse—her lips thin and tight—I knew that it wasn't a time for conversation. I'd seen her like this before, when things were spinning out of control, not going according to plan, as if her stiffness could still the world. She got out of the car, crossed the driveway and climbed the tall set of stairs. She knocked twice, then entered. I heard her yelling at someone, but her voice was the only one I could hear.

"Raymond, please," she begged. "Please come home."

Whether he really wanted to come back or not probably didn't matter. Ray had an iron-clad will and a stubborn streak. And someone was apparently backing him up.

"Stay out of this!" Mom yelled. "He's my son, you stay out of this!"

A short time later she emerged from the house without my brother. She hurried down the stairs and got back into the car. I watched her from the passenger seat as she took off her glasses and wiped the tears from her cheeks, her chin trembling. She took a deep breath, started the car and turned it around in the driveway. She slowly approached the street at the bottom of the driveway and brought the car to a stop, waiting for an opening to enter the sparse but fast-moving traffic. Her eyes still on the road, she spoke aloud, but only half to me.

"My kids come first," she said. "I'd do anything for my kids."

"I know, Ma," I answered.

She turned and looked at me. "You know that we'll always have each other, right?" she asked.

"I know, Ma," I answered.

Her pale-blue eyes still red, she lingered on me a moment longer. Then she returned her gaze to the road on the other side of the windshield. She spotted an opportunity in the traffic and pressed the gas pedal hard to the floor. The wheels spun for a moment, kicking up ruts in the gravel behind us as we sped away. Then we were gone, and so too was Raymond.

RAY WENT to live with my father after that.

Dad still lived back at the ancestral Henick house atop Blueberry Hill, under the shadow of the radar base. Two of his brothers still lived there too. And Nana Marg still reigned with a smoke-filled fury. Nothing changes if nothing changes. Dad was still officially with Joanne, concurrent with a rotating cast of other women, but he had a strict curfew for when he had to be at her house on the appointed evenings. I visited him occasionally, but never in the evening, since that conflicted with her schedule. While Joanne was strict with Dad, my father was much less strict with my brother. My father wasn't ill-intentioned, but he wasn't exactly parent-of-the-year material when it came to firm boundaries and positive role modelling. Raymond later likened living with my father at Nana Marg's house to living in a boarding house. Everyone locked their bedroom doors, and he was surrounded once again by tension and turmoil. Raymond had always been a good student, but after moving in with my father, he stopped going to school.

Gary wasn't a bad person either. He was damaged, no less emotionally than neurologically. Under it all, as hard as it was for me to access or admit, he still had a softness, a generosity that only a few people ever saw. It didn't excuse his behaviour, but it made it less mysterious. Gary was complex, I started telling myself, to help me sleep at night. He certainly wasn't always the cause of every difficulty. Life was still hard, for everyone, after all. Outside the home, he still stood up for us when we needed him. He probably had more opportunities to stand up and defend Krista, because she got herself into difficult situations more often than most people. Her attitude got her in trouble a lot.

She had gone to her Catholic school one morning with a penis-shaped key chain affixed to her backpack. When her English teacher caught her laughing about it with her friends, he instructed her to "put her dildo away" and to play with it at home. She exploded in anger and embarrassment in front of the class and was sent to the principal's office. Krista argued with the old nun, who had been running the school since Mom was a student there. "You need to loosen up, sister," my sister eventually said. "Maybe you should go home and masturbate."

Krista was immediately expelled from Holy Angels High School.

Mom begged, and Gary used his charm, to get Sister Agnes to take Krista back. It mostly worked. Krista could return, but not until the following semester. After that, Gary constantly reminded her to be grateful for what he had done for her. He reminded us all, a lot, about how much he did for us. Especially Mom. By Gary's account, she was desperate and on the rebound before Gary came along to save the day, and it didn't matter that we all saw it the other way around.

Combined with my sister's academic struggles and a lot of missed time, the expulsion ended up delaying her graduation by a year. She was bitter that she wouldn't be able to graduate with her friends.

She and Gary fought often, and most of their arguments ended the same way.

"You're not my father!" she'd scream, her eyes bulging and her round face flushed, hardly an inch from Gary's nose. Then she'd stomp off to her room and slam the door. I envied her ability to stand up for herself, because I so rarely did.

Krista was a fighter.

ONE SUMMER afternoon, Gary orchestrated a teenage fist fight down by his tool shed.

It wasn't spontaneous, nobody had asked for or instigated it, it was just something that he got into his head to do. He brought me, his son Matt and my cousin, who was also named Matthew, back to a small clearing between the birch trees. We were all around the same age, but I was the youngest by a year or so. He explained what was about to happen.

"You think you're so strong?" Gary asked us. Apparently, he had decided that someone had threatened his family's manliness. "See if you can take my Matt."

My cousin and I looked at each other, trying to understand what he was asking of us. Then he clarified.

"Fight!" he suddenly announced.

I was having none of that. I avoided conflict whenever possible. I backed away, stepping up onto the concrete slab where we shot twenty-one in the basketball hoop mounted on the side of the tool shed. Gary glanced sidelong at me but didn't seem to care. I never got the impression he thought much of me. He was fixated on his real son, grinning.

Matt and my cousin looked at each other, shrugged, smiled a little, then seemed to approach it as a game. They began circling each other. My cousin, wiry and a bit awkward, had his hands raised but open and limp at the wrists. He reminded me of something between a dancing monkey and a praying mantis. Gary's son—my stepbrother, as I wasn't entirely opposed to calling him—had a stockier build. He worked out at the gym often and religiously watched wrestling on television. He moved around less and held his hands like the martial artists he played in *Mortal Kombat* games.

They each dodged a few playful swings. Then, moving quickly, Matt clipped my cousin on the left shoulder with a stiff right jab. I could tell it hurt by the way he winced, but my cousin looked more surprised than anything. Gary appeared thrilled. Matt swooped in again. He came in low, and I knew that the next step was supposed to be to wrap his arms around my cousin's torso. He would then pick him up and slam him to the ground. I'd seen him use the move before.

Before Matt could engage, my cousin met his forward motion with a quick, hard slap across his right cheek. It was hard enough to echo between the birch trees and send Matt recoiling back. The side of his face turned an instant, angry red and his eye watered. A swollen white outline of the five fingers and palm that had made full contact with his face started to appear. He touched his cheek lightly with the tips of his fingers and quickly pulled them away again. He looked as though he was fighting with himself not to cry. My cousin stepped forward a little, out of uncertain concern. Gary stepped between them.

"That was a dirty hit!" he protested. "You fight like a girl!"

My stepbrother looked to his father, then jumped back into the fight more fiercely. He tackled my cousin to the ground and they rolled around on the low-cut grass. They tussled and flailed in the dirt for a few frenzied minutes, but it didn't look to me as if either was very focused anymore.

"Okay, that's enough," Gary said, breaking them up. He looked at my cousin and admonished him again, as if knowing his son had lost but seeking to rationalize it. "You're a dirty fighter."

That's how a lot of the fights at Gary's house went, especially when his first family were visiting. It was as though he got a taste of what he'd lost, or suddenly believed that his dreams for them all to come rushing back home were being fulfilled, so there was no need for the pesky Henick replacements anymore. His real family always outranked us. I felt the game was rigged against me and my mom, and from the beginning we were never intended to win.

Mom fought back occasionally anyway, more at first, but with years and maybe age she became more selective in her battles. When she did stand up for herself, one of Gary's standard attacks was to remind her that she was replaceable. That was her greatest weakness. She was learning independence, but she was still vulnerable and lacked self-confidence.

At some point Krista caught on and defended our mom by turning it back on him. "You know I can get rid of you any time I want, right?" she said to Gary with a smile, in the middle of another meaningless fight.

"You think so, do you?" he asked. "How would you do that?"

"It'd be easy," she answered. "You're always talking about how you could get another woman. Next time you're not home, I can just go down to the laundry room and put a condom in your pocket." My mother had had a hysterectomy after I was born. Krista knew she had made her point. "Mom will find it," she said, just to make sure. "Then it's bye-bye Gary."

"You wouldn't dare," he threatened.

"Try me," my sister replied.

Things seemed to simmer down after that. They fought all the time, and there didn't appear to be any love lost between them, but they had an unusual respect for one another. Ironically, in Krista, I think Gary had met his match. She was tougher even than his boys. Krista was only nineteen and still trying to finish the high school credits she needed to graduate. She was bitter that she didn't get to do it with her friends, but she was determined to finish. She was also seven months pregnant. Krista's relationship with Gary seemed to settle more as she became more visibly pregnant. Still, she refused to raise her child in his house. Even though they were on better terms, Gary wasn't about to try to stop her leaving. It would mean another Henick gone. Krista got a little basement apartment with her boyfriend across town.

By early summer, my sister had finally completed the remaining credits that she needed to graduate from high school. On the day of her long-awaited graduation, however, she went into labour. The birth was difficult, with complications and medical errors. Mom was by her side in the delivery room the entire time and helped my sister through the long recovery. It was her first grandchild, and she was so proud of my sister's determination. Against Krista's feigned indifference, Mom went down to her school and picked up the green graduation hat and tassel that she would have worn. She kept it in the box with the picture of me in my bright-red vest and black tie, Raymond's wooden race car, her first nursing name badge and her other most cherished memories, nearly all of which had something to do with our first family.

Krista gave birth to a healthy little boy. It felt weird being a twelve-year-old uncle. All my scores of uncles were much, much older. It also felt weird that my mother was now a grandmother. She shared some of Nana Ag's features but looked nothing like her, and she bore no similarity whatsoever to Nana Marg. However, having become a grandmother so young—and she repeatedly reminded everyone how young a grandmother she was—my mother seemed to revel in the sudden change of status. Something small changed in her, some trigger switched for the very first time. Maybe it was something about how, for all our differences, there was at least one indisputable thing that everybody in our mishmash family could agree on.

Grandmothers were important.

CHAPTER 5

WITH RAYMOND AND KRISTA BOTH GONE, IT WAS just me, my mom and Gary, as well as whichever of his rotating cast of kids happened to be back. Mom tried to leave next.

My mother and Gary had been together for about five years by then. Mom never had much confidence that she could make it on her own, that she could live without a man in her life to support her and control her. I don't think she realized that she had already raised three kids, essentially as a single parent. It was hard, but hard was okay, and she did it through grit and determination. She woke up each morning before dawn and pulled herself out of bed in order to support her kids. There was no other option, she just put her head down and got it done.

She had all but begged Gary to set a wedding date ever since he proposed, but it was becoming clear as the years went by that he had no intention of marrying her. It was in part the promise of marriage that made her stay, the hope that someday things would be better. However, after her first grandchild was born, I think she started to feel more confident, and that she didn't have to wait for somebody else to make her life meaningful. Maybe my mother started to realize that she was going to leave a legacy regardless. With her kids growing up, moving out, having kids of their own, maybe she realized she could be an independent woman after all. That's when she really started trying to leave.

One August day, just after noon, Mom and I rushed down the concrete walkway to the car in the driveway. We were making our escape from the house at the end of the dead-end dirt road, from the fields and forest, from the silence and the screaming. Gary and my mom had been fighting all morning. It was the first of many times that she would try to leave.

"Get back in the house, you crazy bitch," Gary shouted from the side step.

Whereas my mom cried when she screamed, Gary smiled.

"No! Fuck you! Fuck you, you fucking bastard!" Mom screamed back.

Her voice was raw, her face red, her cheeks, lips, brow trembling, her eyes filled with tears. She put her bag in the back seat. I stood at the passenger side door, watching as usual, my own bag already in the car.

"I will never step foot in this house again," she swore. I'm not sure that any of us believed her.

"What time is it, Brenda?" Gary asked.

She didn't answer, she just glared.

"Twenty minutes," he pronounced. "Give me twenty minutes and I'll have someone else in here to replace you," he said. Gary repeatedly worked that weak spot, her lack of faith in herself, her replaceability.

Mom seethed, hurt. "Good!" she finally screamed back.

She ordered me into the car, got behind the wheel and slammed the door. She started the car, jammed it hard into reverse and sped backwards up the long driveway between the big concrete light posts. Shifting into drive, she looked up. Gary was standing on the walkway, at the bottom of the steps. As she reached her arm past me, I felt the heat emanating from her skin. She got her hand as close to the window on my side as possible, then she gave Gary the middle finger and drove off.

Gary never did get another woman, on this escape or any of the ones that came after.

Whenever we left, Gary himself never seemed to change, but something in his house would alter instead. There'd be a different one of his kids visiting, or he'd be working on some new landscaping project on his property, or he'd be remodelling some room in the house, usually in the basement. Fix the foundation—maybe that will change things. He always talked about raising the house a few feet, to get more headroom down there, but he never did. As I got taller, I could easily touch the ceiling when I stood in the basement. I had at least four different bedrooms in that little basement, as Gary kept moving the walls, readjusting the boundaries each time we left and returned, left and returned.

We stayed at Nana Ag's house. She had one of her many little Biblical-passage decorations on the bedroom wall. It was from the Parable of the Wise and Foolish Builders. *The rain fell, the floods came, and the winds blew and buffeted the house,* it read. *But it did not collapse; it had been set solidly on rock.*

The little framed picture didn't mention the part about the fool who built his house on sand.

We went back to Gary's after a few days.

WHEN I CHANGED schools to start seventh grade, from South Bar to Whitney Pier Memorial Junior High School, I also entered the French immersion program. I had liked learning French in grade six. There was something attractive to me about having a language all to myself at home, where nobody else understood it. I did well in my hour-long lessons, so I expected it to be much the same when I switched almost exclusively to French. I was wrong.

It was too much change all at once. It was like a whole different world from the one I knew. I didn't know any of the teachers, and the school was much bigger than my last one. South Bar had one central hallway, while Memorial had four floors, with a loop of hallway around each, and classrooms on both sides. I didn't know anybody outside the school who spoke French, other than my aunt Pat on Mom's side, but I had way too many aunts and uncles to be close to all of them. I didn't understand any of the work. It felt as if I'd been parachuted into a foreign country where I couldn't navigate or communicate, and I had nowhere to turn.

However, it wasn't all bleak. My homeroom teacher was young and pretty. She seemed to like me. I sure liked her. I liked how nice she was to me. I liked how she seemed to actually listen, how she looked me straight in the eyes when she spoke to me. I liked how her blouse clung to her body, illuminated by the sun through the window, as she wrote on the blackboard. Apparently, in addition to my new school, in a new language, I was also entering into a new kind of awareness of the people around me. I was especially starting to notice more of the girls and women in my proximity.

Things seemed to slowly adjust at school as I started to build some routines. However, the situation at home was still hard. With my brother and sister gone, and the occasional flight into exile with my mother, it was hard to find any balance. At home I felt isolated, guilty, shameful, unwelcome yet trapped and, increasingly, unsafe.

These feelings never having been resolved as they developed over the years, they continued to grow wider and deeper inside me.

I didn't dare invite friends over to the house because I had no idea what Gary might say or do to them. I couldn't risk the social cost. What if people went back to school and spread word that my dad—as he was inevitably called before I issued a quick correction—had made them pick rocks from the field or chop wood or fight each other or some other weird competition of manliness. I was insecure, as though my feet were always on sand and I had to be ready for any possible attack. Not all my worries were entirely irrational. I just couldn't tell which ones were.

At the beginning, I felt safer at my new school than I did at home. As had happened when I went to South Bar, I slowly started to move from fear of the unknown to seeing the school as a refuge, a safe space. Over the first few weeks I grew close to a couple of teachers, especially Mrs. Marmulak and Mrs. Walsh. I felt they took the time and effort to look at me tenderly, without judgment or contempt. I believed they saw some of the real me that I was learning to hide inside. They both mentioned having kids with special needs at one point, so maybe that had something to do with their capacity for kindness.

However, the process was interrupted when I started to attract some new bullies.

I was at my locker one day after school when one of them cornered me. He'd been threatening me for a few weeks, but he never made time to stop and introduce himself, so I didn't know his name at the time. I later learned that it was Allen. Allen and some of his gang had taken to waiting for me outside the school, so I often stayed inside long after the last bell to avoid encountering them. I didn't expect him ever to confront me inside. I was tall, but he was taller. Allen was also heavier, faster and stronger than me.

He found me in the half-level basement—the Pit, we called it— where the main bank of lockers was located. He rushed at me, like a charging bull, and we collided straight-on. I hit the line of tall metal locker doors behind me hard. A crowd descended immediately on hearing the crash that echoed through the Pit. "Fight, fight, fight, fight!" the other students chanted in rabid unison.

I bounced back toward him, or propelled myself at him out of blind instinct, I'm not sure. I saw my arm shoot out in front of me. I wasn't thinking, for a change, and in a rush of adrenalin I grabbed him by the throat. He grabbed me with both hands by the front of my shirt. I thought of the way Gary had held Raymond and pinned him against the wall, of the way my brother had writhed and flailed. I squeezed my fingers closed as hard as I could. I felt my nails sink deep into the soft tissue on either side of his Adam's apple, and as I did, I locked him in direct eye con- tact. Eye contact normally made me extremely uncomfortable, as though people could see my secrets behind my eyes, but not this time. His brown eyes bulged, big and round. His lips sputtered and gasped, revealing his clenched teeth, but he wouldn't let go. Neither did I. We held each other close, locked together for what felt like an eternity, but it was probably only a few seconds. He was growling, or choking, and his olive skin started to blush a deep red. I kicked him once, hard, in the stomach. He should have protected himself, Gary would have said if he'd been watching.

Allen jerked away sharply. He let go of my shirt and shoved me back. I rushed forward, intending to kick him again, but I missed. I saw the vice-principal pushing through the crowd that encircled us. He was tall with a white beard and owl-like eyes, and he was shouting for us to stop. Just before he got to us, though, Allen wound up and sent one speeding bulldozer punch directly toward my head. Laser focused in full self-defence mode,

I weaved only a degree or two to the right. His fist whizzed past my left ear and crashed into the locker behind me, denting the aluminum door and sending another loud echo reverberating over the noise. The crowd roared louder. My ears were ringing.

The vice-principal arrived a moment later and broke us up. He asked if I was okay. I don't remember what I said. As the vice-principal escorted Allen by the arm through the parting crowd and out of the Pit, Allen jerked away from him and punched one more locker on the way, sending a last crash echoing through the space. I finally jumped, startled. The crowd thinned and dissipated quickly, and everything became silent. All I could hear was my heart pounding in my ears.

I must have collected myself and got the bus home, as I always did, but there's a gap in my memory. When my awareness came back, I had gotten off the bus and was walking down Gary's long driveway. I continued past the house, to the very end of the gravel in the clearing around the bend. I went down the grassy path into the woods, to the wall of trees. I didn't stop this time, I didn't retreat back to the house, I pushed through the leafy barrier without hesitation. The ground was rough, but I went slowly, careful to navigate around the fallen branches and little hills, over the boggy valleys and slippery moss. It was hard at first but became easier once I got used to the terrain. I didn't know where I was going, I just went. My instinct was to run, to hide, to disappear forever.

As I went deeper into the woods, I heard a trickle of water. I came to a little embankment and climbed to the top. On the other side was a shimmering brook, a tiny flowing stream no more than ankle-deep in some places, knee-deep in others. It wound a thin thread through the trees, escaping from sight in both directions. I sat down on the embankment. I could finally breathe again. Under a dappled canopy of leaves, I watched the water.

This water had somewhere it was supposed to go, I thought. It didn't have some supernatural consciousness, it didn't have to think at all; it just collected itself and carved an ever more certain rut in the earth as it went, getting faster when it rained and deeper over time. It could no more escape its destiny than I could. I studied the stones that sat beneath the crystal water. If they had ever been jagged, broken free from a larger form in the eroding embankment, here they were now, under the water, in the middle of the woods, smooth and round. They had been worn and shaped by the current, all the loose sand around them carried away, and still they were rock.

I noticed the sun. I felt the warmth shine through the leaves above me, on my shoulders, then, when I looked up, the sun on my face. I closed my eyes. I carved each small detail into every sense memory so that I could take it with me wherever I went. All I had to do was close my eyes again and I could feel the sun and the earth, smell the pine and moss, hear the trickling water and see the stones. I'd rather be there than anywhere else, even if only in my mind. I could escape here, to this special place in my head, and be safe. This place understood me in a way I didn't yet know I needed to be understood.

When I opened my eyes, the sun had gone behind a cloud and the woods were darker. I noticed the cool breeze from which the warm sun had distracted me. I watched a leaf blow free from a treetop above, float down toward me, land on the water and be swept away.

The leaf was orange. I looked around and noticed that a lot of them were. I felt a sense of hopeless dread.

I didn't know how I hadn't seen it before.

Summer was over.

PART TWO

THE FALL

A final flood of colors will live on
As my mind dies,
Burned by my vision of a world that shone
So brightly at the last, and then was gone.

—CLIVE JAMES, "JAPANESE MAPLE"

Chapter 6

"YOUR FATHER CALLED HERE," GARY SAID. "HE CALLED your mother a fat pig."

It was a familiar line of attack. He often told me of the nasty things my father apparently said about my mother. It was probably true; it sounded like something Dad would say, but I didn't know why Gary needed to tell me. The comments seemed to come after I had been visiting with my father, which I did off and on, depending on how well he and I were getting along at any given time. Sometimes I felt my dad didn't want me around. He had made it clear that his partner, Joanne, certainly didn't want us around. The feeling was mutual. For Krista, Ray, me and Mom, she was always the Other Woman. Dad saw us anyway, but only when she wasn't around.

Before he made his fat pig comment, I had been telling Gary about a nice visit I'd had with my father. Dad and I had gone fishing. We had started doing that occasionally, but all we ever caught was one emaciated little silver trout. My dad had shown me how to carefully remove the hook from its lip, standing on the rocky lakeshore in the summer afternoon sun. Some days I wondered if Gary wanted to have those moments with me too—or if I wanted them with him—and some days I think he tried. Then there were the other days, most days, when I wasn't convinced he even liked me.

"Why don't you just go and live with your dad?" Gary asked, with the smile that wasn't happy.

I had a nice visit with my father that day, and I felt happy. I could still feel happy sometimes. But then Gary made it seem as if my feelings were wrong, that I shouldn't have seen my dad, and that it shouldn't have been nice. I felt as though, in his quest to regain his former life, Gary was trying to finish off the last of the Nazi Henicks that had infested his house. I felt unwelcome there, inconvenient, increasingly a burden to him. He got the woman, but she came with baggage—her children—and that somehow pissed him off.

I hated feeling I was an inconvenience all the time, an unwanted tagalong. I couldn't carry that weight in my mind forever. So, when I was twelve years old, I started thinking about hurting myself.

I had made it through the first semester and half of the second semester of seventh grade more or less intact. Although the school had only three grade levels, there were half a dozen or more classes at each level. When I told my mother that I had been assigned to 7F, she asked if "F" meant I was failing. I tried to explain that it was because I was in French immersion, but I'm not sure she understood. Being in the youngest cohort, even if only temporarily, also meant I was at the bottom of the hierarchy in the school. Now I was isolated and insignificant again.

I began to have trouble sleeping, and I had a hard time focusing in class. I fell behind slowly at first, then cumulatively when

I couldn't catch up. I think I hid it well enough that nobody noticed at first. If anyone did notice, they didn't say anything. If they did say anything, I didn't hear it. "Don't let them see your weakness," I thought. "Be a man."

The weak get left behind, the weak get eaten alive and forgotten. Over time my fears and anxieties, my insecurities and beliefs about my own worth had become more ingrained in me and had taken root. They were less something I felt and increasingly something I was.

My mother had gone to work before I woke up one day, before the morning sun breached my basement window and slashed across my face. In the darkness of my room, I hated the violent light. I had been fighting with Gary about a board game the night before. We were playing Trouble. We played Trouble a lot. On the last pop of the die, enclosed in its little dome in the middle of the board, Gary rolled enough to get his last plastic marker the rest of the way around. I didn't mind losing, normally, except this time Gary had bet me a hundred dollars that he would win. Being a competitive twelve-year-old, I agreed, and all through the game I was thinking about how I'd spend all that money. That was a lot of money to me, and Gary knew I had about that much saved up from Christmas. About twenty minutes into the game, it became clear that I was about to lose my savings.

When Gary won, he took the money, as we had agreed. It was probably a good life lesson, but I whined. I pestered him all evening to give it back, or at least to play again. I even continued to mention it the next morning. Maybe he hadn't slept well, or he woke up as the Other Gary that morning, or I had just worn him down. I'm sure my nagging must have been irritating. That was the point, after all. So, in my mind, it was my fault that it set him off.

"Be a man," he said in the loud, charged voice. "Lose like a man."

He stomped out of the kitchen, into the red living room that we were rarely allowed to enter. Regretting that I had pushed him too far, I went to the porch to put my shoes on, since the school bus would be coming soon to meet me at the end of the dead-end dirt road. A minute later he was back, marching across the kitchen. His big fists were balled up at his sides when he stopped and met me at the door.

"You want your money?" he said. "Here." He raised one fist and shoved it forward.

I flinched, then saw that he had two fifty-dollar bills clenched between his thick fingers. He was giving me what I had been asking for. Except, after all that, I suddenly didn't want it anymore. I felt guilty after the show he had put on, the way he complained and the spite with which he gave in. I regretted pestering him, acting like such a whiny little girl about it. "Be a man," I thought.

"No, Gary," I said. "Never mind."

"Take your fucking money," he answered.

Before I could say any more, he grabbed my left hand with his hand that was short a finger. He pressed the bills hard into my palm and released me. Then he shoved past me, put on his shoes and went out in the yard to work. There was grass to cut, rocks to pick, lots of things to fix. He slammed the door behind him. In the sudden silence of the back porch, the sound of the slamming door buzzed in my ears. After a few minutes I followed him, ashamed of myself for making him so angry.

The school bus had come and gone, and with Mom at work, I had no other way to get to school. It was too far to walk and I had a test to write that morning.

I hated Gary sometimes. Other times, I hated myself for

hating him. I needed him. I hated that I needed him. My head was increasingly being taken over by hate, at first for others.

Then the hate turned inward.

I SAT in the awkward silence of his big red pickup truck while Gary drove me to school. He didn't speak the entire way. Over the course of the ten-minute drive, partly over the cratered Tank Road, I felt as though my mind was falling under anaesthesia while the rest of me stayed awake. Such a small needle the anaesthetist uses, to alter someone's state so completely. I didn't know what was happening to me. I could feel, but I was numb; I could see, but my vision was narrow; I could hear, but voices sounded slow and slurred. It was as if my brain was shutting off. I had liked to float away in my imagination before, escaping to the image of the stream in the woods that I had planted in my inner world. But this was new.

Gary pulled the truck up to the curb near the main doors of the school. I got out and he drove away without a second glance. I went inside to my locker in the Pit, fiddled with it for a few seconds and got frustrated that I couldn't remember the combination. I had used it hundreds of times before, at least four times a day, every day, but the combination had been completely erased from my mind. Intermittent memory loss had been happening more often lately. It happened when I was feeling a lot inside, and even more often when I was feeling a lot but showing nothing at all on the outside. Sometimes the fog was so thick that, when I came out of it, I could hardly remember where I was or how I had gotten there. It was like I just blacked out for a while.

I got up to Mrs. Ivanov's classroom on the fourth floor, never having gained access to the books in my locker, but the period was almost over anyway. The class of twenty or so grade seven students were sitting quietly at their desks, finishing the test that I was late for. The classroom seemed unusually full and cramped, it felt like the walls were closing in on me. When Mrs. Ivanov saw me from her big desk in the corner, she gestured for me to come over.

"Why are you late?" she asked, in French, without a hello. Her black hair was almost buzz-cut short, her features sharp and angular. She was young, quick and intimidating.

"I'm sorry," I replied. I really was. "I missed my bus."

Her hard stare pierced me. Then she looked at her watch, clucked as if to sarcastically wish me good luck and handed me a clean copy of the test. I took the stapled stack of three or four double-sided sheets and found a place at a desk near the middle of the collapsing, claustrophobic room. I pulled a pencil from my bag and looked down at the test. My mind was blank. I couldn't think. I couldn't remember the answers, couldn't remember if I'd even known them in the first place. I couldn't remember how I got to school. There seemed to be a lot of noise around me. The other kids sat silently, but it sounded in my head as if everyone was talking at once.

The test shouldn't have been a big deal, but it was. If I didn't do well, I always felt it was a personal catastrophe. Meeting people's expectations was important to me, and yet I was failing. I felt dumb and useless at home and at school, and this situation just proved to me that my feelings were justified.

I stared blankly at the page for about five minutes, then spent the remaining ten minutes drawing in the margins. I drew ten different ways I could kill myself. I needed an escape, but imagining myself at the stream in the woods with the sun on my face wasn't enough anymore. If I couldn't find a place to feel safe, outside or inside my mind, then I had to kill myself. Absent other salient options, it was my only choice. There's an internal logic to irrationality.

My inward, downward spiral was interrupted by the ringing of the bell. The remaining ten minutes of the class had passed. "That was quick," I thought. Even time travel was possible when I slipped away. I sat for a while longer at my desk as people got up and left. I felt like a second-grader again, getting a big zero on my test and breaking down in tears. Except this time I couldn't cry and be comforted—certainly not when I was surrounded by my peers, and definitely not with this teacher. The social cost would be too great.

When most of the others were gone, I handed in the test and went back to my desk. It was a double period that morning, so our next class was in the same room. After the short break came the bell, and the class filled up again.

Mrs. Ivanov assigned a reading to start, then called me out into the hall. It was about my margin notes, she said. She had the test in her hand, and she asked what the drawings were. Her tone sounded accusatory, but that may have been just how I was hearing everything. In any case, it certainly didn't sound warm.

"Is this a man blasting off in a rocket?" she asked. She was pointing to one of the little inch-high graphite doodles. It was a stick-figure version of me, dead, hanging by my neck from a tree. The tree was one of the big pines outside the house, beyond the end of the dead-end dirt road, beyond the fields and grassy path, beyond the stream in the forest, where nobody would find me.

I explained to her what it was supposed to be, and we went through some of the others too. Some were unique, others variations on a theme. Hanging, jumping, cutting, stabbing, shooting, drowning, falling, flaming, choking and poison. It was an aimless scattershot, a creative inventory of whatever came to mind. I had no specific intention to do any of them; that part was still vague. It was a suicide brainstorm.

I was embarrassed, not just because she had discovered my secret but also because of my less than perfect drawing skills. "I can't do anything right," I thought. My thoughts had become routinely dark and variably distorted, depending on the circumstances. My thoughts more or less connected to one another, and seemed to make sense to me, but I had no way of knowing if my logic had been skewed by the distorted way in which I had started seeing the world. I saw the world, and all the mounting threats within it, through the only brain I'd ever had—shaped as it was by the environment imposed upon it. If an idea appeared in my thoughts, then I thought the idea must also be true. Dark was normal, normal must be true, therefore dark was true. I wanted to escape my true dark, but I had no idea how it'd ever get better. In the dawn of my seeping depression, this didn't seem like distorted reasoning. It all made perfect sense; everything fit together logically within the frame of logic I was using.

My teacher, apparently, didn't operate within the same logic. She didn't tell me if what I had done was right or wrong. She just sent me to the guidance counsellor as soon as he was available to see me.

Mr. Nichols met with me in his tiny office by the library. It looked like a repurposed walk-in closet—maybe ten feet across in both directions. There was a steel-framed chair by the door, a desk along the wall and a messy bookshelf across from the desk. It wasn't disorderly, but it was obviously occupied by a man more concerned with function than form. Mr. Nichols himself was notably tall, maybe in his early forties. He had a few wisps of grey in his dark hair, but he still came across as young. He was approachable and spoke with a warm, gentle voice. He asked me what was going on. He had my drawings in front of him.

I tried to pass the whole situation off as a reaction to stress, because I had only fifteen minutes to complete the test. I felt that my academic struggles would be more in his wheelhouse anyway, compared with whatever the hell was going on in my mind. I wasn't even close to understanding what was going on in there. He said that he understood I was stressed but that most people don't draw pictures like the ones I drew after they're late for a test. I hadn't really thought about that. I didn't know what was normal for "most people"; I only knew what I knew. He asked me if I had been thinking about hurting myself.

"Yeah," I answered.

He asked me if I had any plans for how I would do it.

"Yes," I said. I walked him through each of the pictures. They weren't plans so much as ideas. I didn't know the difference.

"Mark, I think that you need to go to the hospital," Mr. Nichols said after we'd been talking for about ten minutes. He said it as the kind of suggestion you'd hear every day—you've got to hear this song, you must try this cake, you need to go to the hospital. It sounded strange to me at first. Then I realized that it wasn't a suggestion at all. Mr. Nichols had a professional responsibility for my safety, he explained, and I needed to go to the hospital in order to be safe. I agreed, but I didn't feel I had any choice.

Mr. Nichols called my mother. He explained what had happened and what needed to happen next. I waited in his office until Mom picked me up and drove me to the hospital. I sat silent, ashamed of myself for breaking her peaceful idyll. I was triaged, and she waited with me in the emergency room, mostly in silence. We sat there for hours before we were finally brought in to talk to the social worker.

12 yr old male into ER accompanied by his mother Brenda, the social worker wrote on the lined notepad that had CRISIS ASSESSMENT printed in bold at the top. *Unknown to mental health services,* she noted below it. In the top corner of the page, she wrote the date: *April 13, 2000.* She asked me the same questions Mr. Nichols had—if I'd been thinking about hurting myself and if I had a plan. I said yes to both. She asked me about the plan and I told her about how I could go into the woods.

"Then you know what would happen," I said, assuming that everyone would understand what I meant. I mean, it was obvious to me, and my thoughts felt like reality, so it must be obvious to others. I think that's why I felt frustrated when she kept asking questions. It was as if I didn't have the language I needed to explain what was going on inside me; I was like a little kid who knows what he feels but can't yet say the words. I wished there was a resource like the French-English dictionary I carried to class every day, but one that translated from my head to my mouth.

I answered all the social worker's questions as best I could. I told her about how little energy I had, how little I'd been eating, how I couldn't concentrate or remember things, how easily I became frustrated and irritated. I told her that I felt worthless, hopeless, sad, guilty and lonely. I told her about how much I cried when I was alone in my basement room with the door closed.

Mom sat next to me and listened. The social worker turned to her and asked her what she had noticed about me. She was quiet for a long time. When she finally spoke, her voice was dry and professional. Most of the time that my mother spent in hospitals, often in twelve-hour shifts, she was the one checking the charts and asking the questions.

"I was shocked," she said. "Mark is quiet and spends a lot of time alone. I guess he's been tired a lot, and he's been having trouble at school." She paused, then finally admitted: "I didn't think it was this bad." Her voice quivered. "I didn't see this coming." She tightened her mouth and her lips drew thin.

The social worker handed her a box of tissues. She took two but didn't use them. She looked at me and I saw what looked like failure in her eyes. Not my failure, but hers. She reached out and held my hand, then turned back to the social worker.

"Mark is a good boy," my mom said.

I spoke with several more people, including, eventually, a doctor. I was released from the hospital with a referral to come back and meet with a Child and Adolescent Services worker in a few days. We had waited in the emergency room for so long that whatever crisis Mr. Nichols thought I was in had long since passed. I was tired and just wanted to go home.

Mom drove back to Gary's. He and Carey were working on some landscaping far down the long driveway, near the little parking area past the tool shed, past the birch trees. She pulled the car up near them and rolled down her window. I sat in the passenger's side seat with my head lowered.

"Where've you been?" Gary asked pleasantly. He was often in a good mood when he was working outside.

"Crisis intervention," Mom answered.

In my memory she sounds annoyed. Gary didn't know what she meant. However, I heard Carey's voice from close behind him. "Oh no," she said. She seemed to have a very good idea what it meant. The immediate result of my first visit to hospital for my mental health was the feeling I'd dreaded most: I had let everyone down.

Good boys aren't supposed to have hard times.

CHAPTER 7

I STARTED THERAPY FOR THE FIRST TIME TEN DAYS before my thirteenth birthday.

My clinical social worker's name was Amy. She was probably in her early thirties, with long, curly brown hair. She was warm and friendly, and I liked her. She had an unpretentious, casual style of conversation that made me feel she was speaking to me as a regular person, not as a patient or student or son. She didn't talk at me as though there were some imaginary glass barrier between us; she just conversed with me directly—which was nice. In our first session together, with my mother sitting at my side, Amy explained to me confidentiality and its limits. She'd have to tell someone, she said, if I was a danger to myself or to others. I was starting to understand that concept better now. It made me a little nervous about being too honest.

We talked about my drawings, my impromptu list of all the ways I had imagined I could kill myself, and I told her about how I'd been feeling. I'd lose my place while reading, and it seemed to take me longer than everyone else to copy things from the board into my notes at school. I felt dumb. I was afraid to raise my hand. Whenever I was called upon to speak in front of the class, it brought on a wave of heat and sweat and an irrepressible desire to bolt from the room. I couldn't sleep at night, but I also couldn't get out of bed in the morning. I felt as if I was caught in purgatory—between Henick and Costigan, Sydney and Whitney Pier, kid and teenager, alive and dead.

I'd been discharged from the emergency room with a diagnosis of major depressive disorder, with a query for social anxiety disorder. Amy said she suspected many of my underlying issues were coming from "problems relating to certain family members," as she put it, but also from my own "need for perfection." She sensed that I put a lot of pressure on myself to do well and to please others.

How did she get inside my head? I hadn't had those words for it, but it felt right. I was a little more hopeful that someone was starting to understand me, or was at least trying. Amy suggested at the end of our hour together that I would benefit from ongoing counselling. I didn't have any objection to that. Mom was agreeable, but she seemed a little more hesitant.

Over the next few months I saw Amy about a half-dozen more times, every week or two. We connected well and it was as though we'd known each other a lot longer. Sometimes my mother joined us, sometimes it was just me. In those sessions, Amy taught me for the first time about the connection between thoughts, feelings and actions, and how each can affect the others. She challenged me to intentionally do at least one thing each week that I enjoyed, and when I did that, she asked me to add a second enjoyable thing. She taught me some positive affirmations—"I am smart" and "I am loved," among others—which I was to repeat to myself as often as possible. We kept a mood diary to track how I was feeling and to talk about changes from session to session. We also developed a crisis plan together, so I would know what to do if I was overwhelmed by my emotions and didn't know where to turn.

I was intensely interested in the work we were doing, because it gave me a way to understand how I was feeling. I believed I was finally learning some practical tools, and this gave me a sense of control over myself. If I could figure my mind out, maybe I could fix it. It didn't make my worries and struggles go away, but it helped me manage them better.

By the time my end-of-year exams approached, I was feeling stressed again. Amy and I had started to discuss the possibility of this happening, so I was a little more aware of it and we tried to prepare. However, coping skills are easier to talk about when you don't have to use them. The first test came in June.

I was sitting in English class. It was a class in which I had been doing reasonably well, compared with my other classes, probably because English was taught in English. At the end of each semester everyone's final exams were all written at the same time in the gymnasium. The floor was covered with thin black protective mats, on top of which sat row after row of desks, hundreds of them, like an army of terracotta soldiers. I could avoid the exam, and that terrifying scene, by obtaining a grade of 80 percent or higher. "Accreditation," as it was called, was probably intended as an incentive to do well. In my still mostly negative mindset, however, I saw it the other way around: writing the exam was a punishment for doing poorly. If you were in that room, it was because you were among the lowly underclass of 0 to 79 percenters. Now, nearing the end of the year, in early June, my English score stood at 78 percent. I had previously felt a little pride in that, because it was by far my highest mark.

My English teacher called me into the hall. She also called on two other students to join us. I got up from my desk and looked at the clock as I walked toward the door. It was about seven minutes before the lunch bell was to ring. When I was scared, I had noticed that I would start to focus on very specific details around me, blocking out everything else. This intense focus helped to ground me, like grabbing on to an anchor point in the present so I didn't wash away. I don't remember if I had learned this technique from Amy or if it came from my own efforts to stay afloat.

When all three of us were in the hallway, the teacher led us to an empty classroom around the corner. She arranged us side by side, sitting on top of the front row of desks. She stood facing us, in front of one of the new whiteboards that all the blackboards had been converted to, leaning backwards against a large table behind her.

"As you all know," she began, "exams are coming up in two weeks."

We sat in silence. Of course we knew that, it was just about all we could think of.

"I brought the three of you in here because you're all very close to getting accreditation," she continued. She looked to the boy sitting two desks to my left. "Michael, you deserve it. You've been trying, and I can see that," she said. He smiled, relieved. She turned to the girl in the middle. "Stephanie, I'm not sure about you," she continued. Stephanie smiled too. "You're going to have to really work hard on this last assignment. If you do, you might be able to make it."

Then she turned to me. My heart skipped and my breath turned shallow. I could already sense the guillotine blade coming.

"Mark," she said. "You don't deserve it. You're not trying hard enough."

That was it, that's all it took. Off with his head. It shouldn't have been a big deal, but triggers can be trivial. Pulling a trigger requires very little, but when all the right criteria are met, it can set off a chain reaction with much bigger consequences.

The bell rang. I pretended I was calm, outwardly accepting her determination as fair and reasonable and well presented. Inside, the needles on my anxiety and self-worth gauges were buried in the red zone, and alarms were blaring from every direction. We got up and walked back to the classroom. The other kids were packing their things and fleeing for lunch, and it was noisy.

I packed up and left the classroom too, but I didn't follow the rush downstairs. Instead, I slowly walked the loop of second-floor hallway with classrooms lining either side. When I got back to where I had started, I was finally alone.

I approached Mr. Nichols's tiny office. I looked behind me to check if anyone was watching, then I went in. It was an instinct. I was deciding from moment to moment what to do. Mr. Nichols had seemed nice, and he had helped me when my drawings attracted the teacher's notice, so when I saw his office, I went in. It wasn't some grand plan; going to him for help was an impulse, just as the drawings had been. The smallest building blocks of habits can be either helpful or destructive, depending on the habit that's being built.

Through the open door, I saw him before he saw me. He was sitting at his desk, long legs splayed awkwardly under it. He was eating a sandwich and looking over some papers. He glanced up as I knocked softly, smiled and greeted me. I stood uncomfortably in his doorway, not entirely certain what to say.

"Can I talk to you?" I asked.

"Sure, come in," he answered.

Since he already knew a bit about the secret life in my head, it wasn't as hard to open up to him as it was with strangers. I sat down and told him what had happened. I was trying my best to use the still-new coping and self-expression skills I had been learning from Amy, but mastering a new language takes time and practice and I was still only on the alphabet. I told him how I felt that the English teacher was right, that I wasn't good enough—at least, that's how I heard it—and how I felt that nothing I ever did was good enough.

Mr. Nichols took time to validate my experience. He said that the way the teacher handled the situation was wrong, and he offered to talk with her about it. Then he asked the question that had probably been on his mind since I walked through his door.

"Are you thinking about hurting yourself again?" he asked.

"Yes," I said. I couldn't just forget my old way of coping. The path into that particular dark wood was a little clearer now than it had been when I was just pushing blindly through the trees on impulse alone. Those kinds of habits also become easier with practice. This way of thinking was still my routine. I'd been working on it, piece by piece, at least since I was five, so it wasn't all going to be undone in a few months of hour-long conversations, however helpful they were.

"I'm trying not to," I added, feeling the need to reassure him. I was remembering things that I liked to do, telling myself that people loved me, distracting myself from the thoughts in my head, and it seemed to be working well enough for now.

Mr. Nichols asked if I would be willing to go in and see my therapist right away. I agreed. At least it wasn't the emergency room again. I didn't want to go back there—it was boring, I had to talk to too many people, it smelled funny, and it wasn't very helpful. He called and was able to set up an appointment with Amy in about an hour's time. Then he called my mother.

I sat at the table in the study area outside Mr. Nichols's office, again waiting for Mom to come and pick me up. When she arrived, he explained the situation and she agreed to take me to my appointment at the hospital. Although my mood was still down and my anxiety was running high, it was all very orderly and efficient. I think that helped my own efforts to regain control. Nobody overreacted. It was easier to anchor myself in the whirlpool of my thoughts when the anchor itself wasn't also spinning.

When I got to Amy's office, I started feeling better almost right away. I felt supported and safe. We talked for a while, and she explained to me how this wasn't a setback. She reassured me that recovery from the kinds of things I was dealing with doesn't usually happen overnight. As we talked it through, I realized that, while some things seemed bad at this moment, overall my situation wasn't as bad as it had been a few months ago. We reviewed my mood charts, which showed that I was improving, and having that proof helped. It was a way to step out from the trees and again see the forest. The graph was bumpy and showed me that my recovery was an ever-evolving average, not an absolute point in time. Overall, outside this one moment, I was feeling better.

However, there was still the issue of wanting to die. Amy was concerned about that.

There appears to be some discrepancy between Brenda's observation of Mark's mood and Mark's reported mood, she wrote in her session notes. She was at least somewhat worried about the growing number of methods and plans for suicide that I seemed to be mentally experimenting with. Suicidal ideation is the visualization of suicide; it's mental practice. Practice builds confidence, and confidence overcomes inhibition. That's what Amy was concerned about, even as I hid it from my mom, and even as I think my mom resisted believing it.

Amy floated the idea of using medication to treat my depression. To explain the need for medication, she drew a picture of what she identified as two neurons. She did it on the whiteboard in her office in red dry-erase marker. There was a space between the two, the synapse, and within the synapse she drew little red circles. She identified those circles as serotonin, floating between the two neurons. I needed more of the little red circles. Medication might help with that. Mom was polite but not enthusiastic about the idea.

"My son doesn't need any mind-bending pills," she said aloud later, as we walked to the car.

To deal with Amy's most pressing concern, she and I drew up and signed a contract in which I promised not to hurt myself. At least for the time being, the contract seemed to hold. I felt good about that. It was a small win, achieved with a lot of guidance and hand holding, but I clung to it.

I passed the test.

AMY EXPLAINED to me that learning to cope with stress and adversity was a lot like learning to ride a bike.

I could understand that. When I was five, I had a purple bicycle. My purple bicycle had training wheels. One Saturday morning when I was visiting my dad at Nana Marg's after he had left us, he decided it was time for my training wheels to come off.

"It's time for you to learn to ride by yourself," he said.

On Sunday morning, after mass at Holy Redeemer, my mother brought me down to Nana Ag's house so I could ride my bike with some of my many, many cousins, while she drank tea with her sisters at the kitchen table.

An older cousin led me up Railroad Street a short way, the steel plant's tall smokestacks watching over us in the distance. He helped me find my balance on the bike, then gave me a big push. I accelerated quickly, and I didn't have time to think. When I realized there were no steadying hands or training wheels to keep me upright, my feet shot out to either side of me. Sure, I should have put them on the pedals, but that wasn't my first instinct. I screamed a long, siren-like scream as I whizzed by Nana Ag's house.

"Mark! Put your feet on the pedals!" I heard someone, maybe my mother, shouting to me from the sidelines. I couldn't, they were spinning too fast by that point. When I came near the end of the street, the overpass looming overhead, I finally dug my heels into the ground. I skidded in a slapstick semicircle, fell off my bike and sprained my wrist.

I learned to ride a bike eventually—but not that day. When I did learn, it was in my own way, at my own pace.

Amy helped me to learn at my own pace, but still with a push, and she coached me through the falls. The work we did together helped me start to understand my thoughts, my feelings, my actions and reactions. The result was that I began to sense I was gaining more control over my life. Maybe I didn't have to be trapped inside myself, a slave to my own mysterious emotions.

I was eager to improve. I practised the basic cognitive behavioural therapy skills that she gave me, I tried to keep on top of my homework, and I started listening to Tony Robbins self-help CDs. I taught myself hypnosis through online courses and played subliminal-message audio tracks while I slept—none of which seemed excessive or desperate at the time. My mom thought most of this was weird, and she mentioned as much to my sister, but my mother didn't stop me from pursuing whatever approach I believed might make a difference. It all seemed to be working.

Doing something—anything—seemed to help. Bad moments, while still bad, seemed to pass.

I made it through the rest of the school year, and summer returned. It was a chance to start fresh. Without the pressure of school or the isolation of being snowed in with Gary, I had more freedom to be myself and do what made me happy. Recovery is easy when it's not so hard. Mom got me an acoustic guitar for graduating class as a reward. That gave me something new to focus on, something to learn and become passionate about, and to occupy my time and thoughts.

Once I began to feel better, it became easier to forget about the supports that helped me to feel better in the first place. I started to miss my appointments with Amy. In August, she called and spoke to my mom. Amy told my mother that she was leaving her position, and she asked if I should be referred to a new therapist in order to continue treatment.

"No," my mother said. "He doesn't need therapy anymore. He's doing much better."

After four months of relative progress, Amy let go of my handlebars and my file was closed. Even though I'd seen her less over the summer, simply knowing that Amy was there if I needed her was reassuring. When I found out she had left, I felt abandoned. Still, the structures we had built together to support my coping stayed more or less standing for about a year.

I did okay, even if not great, through eighth grade. Christmas came and went, my fourteenth birthday, and even the end-of-year exams. I achieved accreditation in two subjects that year, so I didn't have to write those exams. Matt came back partway through the year. He didn't go to school much and stayed through the summer. Gary and my mother hadn't been fighting much that year; when it was just us at home, that was more often the case.

After Matt came back, they started fighting more, and we briefly moved out again. Mom had another of her seizures while we were between homes. After her brief hospitalization, we returned to Gary's. She wasn't allowed to drive for a while after that, so ended up even more dependent on him. I started hanging out more with Matt and his friends, since they were all around the house so much, and he and I usually got along well.

"You're like his little sidekick," one of his friends said to me in the side porch one evening. It was after the most recent time that Mom and I had left and come back. His friend wasn't saying it to be funny; she was saying it to be mean. She made that clear. It made me realize how small and desperate I had already been feeling. Maybe I'd been hanging around them too much, I thought, especially since I had started to feel lonelier again and wanted to be around people more.

The same girl asked me to take her to her eighth-grade prom. I did, and when I picked her up, she made fun of how I had styled my hair. She continued to tease me until we got to the school where the prom was held, and the teasing finally became too much. I felt the sudden urge to stand up for myself. So I left her there, simply turned around and walked out. She screamed from the doorway for me to stop, but I didn't even look back. I walked five kilometres home in the middle of the night, and it felt good.

That summer, however, I got a concussion playing soccer. Focusing on the ball, I collided with the head of another player, knocking myself out cold. When I woke up, dizzy, there was a small group of people around me and they carried me off the field. I don't remember how I got home, but I slept for at least three days after. Nobody took me to the hospital.

I spent much of the rest of the summer by myself, since Mom worked and Matt was still playing soccer or hanging out with his friends. Gary hardly came in from tending to his landscape when the weather was nice, and he had accepted a number of logging jobs that took him away a lot. I felt estranged from everyone.

As the summer came to an end and fall approached, my sleep started to get worse. I gradually lost my appetite. My feelings of loneliness and sadness and fear started to creep back, like old friends returning from a long retreat.

Then, the night before the first day of ninth grade, I had a dream.

I'm riding in a school bus. I must have gotten on at the end of the driveway, by the big concrete light posts at the end of the dead-end dirt road. There's field and forest on three sides. The fourth side, the direction the road returns, is the only way out.

I'm alone. The air is thick and warm. I'm seated about a third of the way back, in the passenger side row of double seats. There's a driver, but I can't see him. I assume he's there since we're moving. Somebody has to be driving the bus.

We reach the other end of the dead-end road. Straight ahead is the cratered Tank Road. To the right is the big hill where Gary ripped off his fingers. To the left is the graveyard with the little green crematorium, no bigger than a shipping container, where it smells like campfire hot dogs when they burn people.

We turn around and go back the way we came. The driver accelerates toward the end of the dead-end dirt road, toward the last house in the woods. We again reach the end of the road, again without stopping, without resting, and again the driver turns and speeds in the opposite direction. He sticks with this cycle, repeating it again and again. With each return I become more afraid. I realize what's happening. I gasp for air.

I'm trapped.

My eyes dart around the bus, through the window to the

passing exterior. My heart races, my face is hot and flushed. All I can do is watch the world on the other side of the glass. "I don't want to do this anymore," I shout. I want to escape the dead-end cycle, but I can't get off at either end.

I look for the driver, desperate, but I can't see him. I notice a figure in the seat in front of me. Another passenger? Has someone been there the whole time?

The figure stands, turns to face me and looks me in the eyes. This stops my heart. It's not human. I stare at its small, gaunt features, its hunter-green leather skin. It smiles a cruel sneer. It speaks in a dark, gravelly voice, not with its mouth but with my own thoughts. Its voice is a voice in my own head.

"You are not the Christ," it says.

I can't breathe.

I woke up from the dream with a gasp. I was shaking and soaked with sweat. I got up and looked out my tiny basement bedroom window.

It was still dark, long before dawn.

CHAPTER 8

ON SEPTEMBER 11, 2001, WHEN THE FIRST PLANE HIT the World Trade Center at 8:46 a.m., I was skipping school for the first time. I was fourteen and had started ninth grade about a week before. I told my mother I was sick. Since nobody was home, I came out of my room and lay on the couch in my pyjamas almost the entire day. At 9:03 a.m., I watched live on CNN as the second plane hit the South Tower. Before both towers eventually collapsed, the images of people jumping from the windows was seared into my mind. Facing certain catastrophe, I thought, people would do things they otherwise could never imagine.

I wasn't in class on that second Tuesday morning of the school year because I had started feeling inside as though I was collapsing too. It was even worse this time than the time before the relative improvement, as though I'd torn off a scab that had only just started to heal. I didn't have any desire to leave the house, so to me that meant I couldn't. In reality—or what we understand as reality—there was no equivalence whatsoever in what happened that morning; but my brain once again processed even the most trivial things as a personal 9/11 inside me—except that now, after experiencing a brief improvement, I felt even worse than before. Everything, everywhere, felt like a threat to my personal safety.

I'd been out of therapy for a year, and I had stayed upright for a little while, but I never really learned how to ride the bike. I was just coasting. Nothing changes, if nothing changes. So I reverted to the mean, the pattern that had been, for me, normal. Routine can cut both ways. So now I was just rolling down the street screaming, still not expecting the crash.

One sunny November morning, my mother and I were going to the mall. She was driving and I was in the front passenger seat. We came to a stop at a red light behind a long line of cars. The car behind us didn't stop. Just before the driver smashed into our trunk at full speed, I was looking out the passenger side window, watching the people at Wendy's eat hamburgers. Then I glanced down at the side mirror and saw the black car speeding toward us from behind. There were two men in their mid-twenties in the front seat. I remember looking directly at the driver's face, as he looked straight ahead. I could swear he was smiling.

My body realized before my mind what was about to happen. My legs stiffened, my knees locked, my feet pushed hard into the carpeted car floor, preparing for impact. I gasped, intending to scream, then froze, still holding the man's face in my sight. An instant later the black car's front end crushed into the back of our car, shattering its front windshield into a million pieces and crumpling the hood like an accordion. During the slow-motion, three-second face-to-face we had in my side mirror, I didn't have time to put my hands up and protect myself.

When he collided with us at full speed, our car was thrust forward and I was momentarily thrown back into my seat. When both cars came again to a sudden stop, my torso wrenched forward while my lower body stayed planted, braced by my locked joints. The connective tissue in my left hip felt like hot Velcro being torn away as my chest folded forward toward my knees. The impact echoed from my hip through my left knee and ankle. The right joints must have been softer or luckier.

We had upgraded from the holey red Pony to a lime-green Hyundai Accent, and we now had the luxury of airbags, but they don't deploy when you're hit from behind. The muscles in my back, in my neck and along my spine, all seemed to sense the bare dashboard coming toward my head. They reacted with a strong counter-motion, slowing me enough to avoid a face full of vinyl. The whole thing lasted only a few seconds.

For months afterwards, driving anywhere in the car was terrifying. There was one S-shaped bend in the road, by the Blockbuster Video, just before a set of train tracks that used to carry coal into the old steel plant. Whenever we navigated around it, even at low speed, I felt my fingernails dig into my thighs so hard that they left marks. I could see the man's smile speeding toward me. That's the thing about triggers—they're rarely the real problem. I wasn't afraid of Blockbuster, or train tracks, or even S-shaped bends in the road. I was afraid of the feeling that, for whatever reason, was momentarily called to mind. One scary moment in a car was overgeneralized to mean that riding in cars was scary.

Resilience is a muscle. I think mine had been exhausted, or atrophied, or never fully developed in a functionally helpful way in the first place. This made it easier for me to get hurt, and harder for me to heal. The pain in my hip, knee and ankle left me off school for weeks, hobbling around on crutches. I fell behind in my school work again, back where it felt I deserved to be, but at least I had what I could claim was a good reason this time. I was having more difficulty than ever in keeping up anyway.

In a follow-up appointment for the injuries experienced in the collision, I told my family doctor how I was feeling. She knew my history, so she decided to prescribe my first antidepressant. I don't think she told me about the black-box warning label it carried, as most antidepressants do. It indicated that the medication might increase the risk of suicidal thinking and behaviour in children and adolescents. One of the various theories is that when this happens, the antidepressants are actually working, they're alleviating the depression, but the depression was serving a self-protective, inhibiting function. Without that inhibition, and with less than effective learned coping mechanisms to fall back on, any underlying suicidality can be unleashed. Prescribing guidelines recommend that, when children are prescribed antidepressants, they should be watched closely, especially for the first four weeks. Worsening symptoms or any unusual changes in behaviour could mean trouble. Nobody was watching me.

The collision left me nervous, afraid, limited and different, but for a new reason. It also gave me a taste of what it felt like when people really cared about something that had hurt me. Now, they could see my crutches and my limp, and they seemed more than willing to accommodate my needs. I was even given the key to the elevator at school, to make it easier for me to get to class and keep a normal routine. I didn't have to ask for help—help was offered. Since I had never really had any significant health issues that were physical, this felt new.

Something inside my mind was breaking, gradually shutting down, and it made me feel as though people didn't care about me. It didn't matter that some people probably did. Mr. Nichols and Amy stood out to me as people who cared, but it wasn't necessarily because of what they did for me. They didn't do much. Rather, it was how they did it. It was how they sat with me, and looked at me, the tone they used when they spoke with me and how I felt when I was around them. As for the doctors and nurses, many of the teachers, even my parents, when they offered help in their own ways, it felt wrapped in blame and inconvenience.

With the exception of a few notable figures, the vast majority of people I encountered were indifferent. Either they didn't notice and so did nothing, or they noticed but didn't care and so did nothing, or they noticed and cared but didn't know what to do and so did nothing. Much later, the indifferent ones became forgettable, but in the moment, their silence was deafening. The silence of the indifferent amplifies the vicious voices of those few who do indeed mean harm. And those were the voices that drew my attention. I was surrounded by faceless, unfeeling villains.

That was probably the result of a combination of two things. First, I was hypersensitive to people's reactions toward me anyway. I read things into words and behaviours that probably weren't intended, and I projected my shame and guilt onto the world everywhere I went. However, how I felt wasn't all my fault. A doctor giving me a medication wasn't helpful on its own, even if that's what a doctor is supposed to do to help. I felt that people didn't fully appreciate the amount of pain and loneliness I felt inside me all the time, because they couldn't see it. To me, it felt as though everyone around me was smiling at my funeral. Most people looked, to me, like cardboard cut-outs of what a caring person is supposed to look like without being the real thing. I couldn't feel their feelings, and that bothered me a lot. Everybody, everything, felt fake. I felt fake.

Maybe it was a logical sequence of developmental events, or maybe something in my brain just changed, I don't know. I noticed it when my leg was injured in the car accident, because something felt different about how people reacted to me. Sure, maybe they asked "How are you doing?" in both cases, checking in on both my emotional and physical pain. But when they saw my crutches, their eyes looked different, their voices sounded different, they appeared less anxious and tense. Less like cardboard cut-outs and more like real people. On crutches, I got the impression people openly cared about my well-being, and I didn't feel they blamed me for my difficulties. Compassion was harder to find when it was my mind that was trying to recover from injury.

I guess my own behaviour made it harder for people to feel compassion for me. I thought I was hard to like. I made mistakes. That wasn't a symptom of my mental illness. My illness wasn't all of me, and it didn't explain my every action. Just like someone who has had a positive, healthy, supported, trauma-free life, I could do nice things and some really shitty things all on my own.

I returned to school in December, and I noticed a girl named Emily. I knew who she was; I had seen her at Holy Redeemer every Sunday. She and her little sister sang in the children's choir, and their mother always sat nearby. Although we had never spoken, I was infatuated with her. She was an angel. She had fair skin speckled with light-brown freckles and long red hair that fell past her waist. She was a year younger than me, and in the grade behind.

I'd been an altar boy since I was about ten, and even through my troubles I still relied on the predictable routine the church provided. Every time I served at morning mass, I spent most of the hour on my stool off to the side of the altar staring out at Emily in the pews. It gave me a reason to look out into the sea of people, at that one place where she always sat, and not be nervous. I always got the sensation she was looking back at me, but then again, especially from the front of the room, I often felt that everyone was looking at me anyway. It was like that painting of Jesus near my Nana Ag's bathroom: wherever you went, including the bathroom, his eyes seemed to follow you.

When I got back to school after the car accident, still on crutches, something had changed in me. Maybe it was the anti-depressants working, or the car accident, or the proper motivation, I'm not sure, but my inhibitions were less. I still didn't have the courage to talk to Emily in person, but a sense of urgency swept over me. I needed to share my feelings.

In the first note I wrote to her—at two or three pages, really more of a letter—I proclaimed my undying love. I described how beautiful she was in my eyes, and how I wished for nothing more than for us to be together. After school, when everyone had gone home, I stayed behind. I hobbled down into the locker pit on my crutches, with the letter in hand. I knew where her locker was because I watched her whenever I was fortunate enough to catch a glimpse. When I noticed that she and her small group of friends hung out by her locker after lunch, I and my small group of friends magically migrated our hangout to the row of benches in the lobby overlooking that part of the Pit. Checking twice to make sure no one was around, I slipped the note into her locker and took off. That was on Tuesday.

The next morning—I always arrived before her—I staked out her locker from my place on the bench overhead. One by one, my few friends arrived and joined me. When Emily got there, she went to her locker, opened it and saw the note fall out. I watched her read it, as casually as possible, so my friends didn't notice. She went through the letter, looked around, appeared to think for a moment and put it in her bookbag. I felt a rush of accomplishment, both because I'd expressed myself fully and honestly, in writing at least, and because I'd successfully executed a covert operation.

In perfect Pavlovian fashion, the payoff for my actions left me wanting more. I wrote the second letter in class. It was less romantic. In fact, it was quite explicit. Now that we were being honest—even if my perspective was a little one-sided—I felt it was time to share all of my fourteen-year-old fantasies. Like the time before, I waited until after school, slipped the letter into her locker and limped away. That was Wednesday.

The next morning, I got to school early and watched. She arrived, went to her locker, opened it and saw the note fall out. She read through it, furrowed her brow a little and put it in her bookbag. The bell rang and we all went off to class.

Just before the start of second period, I was on my way to English class when I saw my teacher, Ms. Singh, in the hallway talking to the principal, Mr. Forbes. Mr. Forbes was a tall man with tanned skin, a moustache and a dark ring of long hair around the back of his head, which was bald and shiny on top. Ms. Singh came into the room and told us we were going to start the day with a small writing assessment. She told us it was nothing to be worried about, it wasn't going to be graded, it was just to check and see how everyone was doing. She wrote a line of text on the board that everyone was to copy down on a narrow slip of paper.

"The quick brown fox jumps over the lazy dog," it said.

She told us specifically that we were to print. I was glad about that, since I'd never gotten the hang of cursive and still avoided using it. I copied down the text, thinking it a strange activity but not entirely unreasonable, and handed it in. The teacher put the stack of writing samples into a big yellow envelope, sealed it, signed the seal and had a student take it down to the office. I was starting to feel uneasy, but I nearly always felt uneasy, so I didn't entirely trust how I felt anymore.

About twenty minutes later, a long, low beep emitted from the intercom speaker in the classroom. Different from the higher, more distant-sounding beep that preceded the school-wide announcements in the morning and afternoon, this one was for direct-to-class communication. Everyone looked at the speaker, as though the voice on the other end could see us.

"Ms. Singh, can you send Mark Henick to the office, please?" the principal said.

My heart skipped. These in-class communications weren't uncommon; usually, it was for somebody who had forgotten their lunch or had to leave for an appointment. The entire class erupted in a collective "Ooooooo," as they did for every such announcement. Ms. Singh hushed them.

"Yes, he's on the way," she replied, then nodded for me to go.

When I arrived, the principal was waiting. I went into his rectangular office, brightly lit by a long window on one wall. He sat at a big L-shaped desk with the long side against the wall under the window. He told me to close the door and motioned for me to sit in one of the two chairs that were arranged at the little arm of the L that jutted out from the wall.

As I sat, I saw the stack of papers on his desk. I noticed right away that they were the writing samples we had handed in. A few had some markings, notes and letters circled in red pen. Mine was on top of the messy pile, and it had a lot of red on it. All at once I knew why I was there. I sat in silence.

"Well, Mark, we have a situation," Mr. Forbes started matter-of-factly. "Another student brought these letters to me this morning," he continued. "I had a look, and based on what's written in them we figured out that they were written by a grade nine

French immersion student. When we compared them to these here samples"—he put his hand on the stack—"we saw that they had a lot in common with yours."

"Yeah," I replied.

There was no sense in denying it. We both knew I did it. I understood the gravity of "the situation," as the principal put it. I was also a little impressed with the depth and speed of his detective skills.

"Now this first letter, well, it's nice enough," he said, picking up the quarter-creased paper with my handwriting in his right hand. "But this one isn't so nice," he went on, picking up the other paper in his left hand.

"No," I replied.

I wasn't really anxious anymore. Anxiety is a future thing. It happens when you're afraid of something that hasn't happened yet, or may never happen at all. This happened. So, instead, I was ashamed. I knew that what I had done was wrong.

"She was pretty upset, Mark," the principal said.

I told him that it wasn't my intention to upset her. Actually, it was the exact opposite. We agreed that the best thing for me to do would be to apologize. I waited as he went back out to call Emily from class down to his office. She arrived a few minutes later, came in and sat down in the chair next to me. I apologized to her, trying to make eye contact with her as much as possible so she knew I was sincere, but I had a hard time prying my gaze from the floor between my feet. I felt guilty because I was guilty. I couldn't attribute my behaviour to any symptom or distorted thinking; I had only myself to blame. I regretted what I did and how I made her feel.

It's what happened next that made things problematic.

My apology, as far as I could tell, seemed to be accepted and to resolve the matter. Still, my mind continued to run with the terrible choices I had made, turning them over again and again, overgeneralizing the situation like I did with my acquired fear of riding in the car, spinning it into something else entirely. I had done a bad thing, but throughout the day that fact was getting filtered through my mind's increasingly pathological pathways to mean that *I was a bad thing.*

Eventually, it wasn't even about the event anymore, it had nothing to do with Emily or the letters or the fact that I got caught. My anxiety rushed back as I imagined my mother finding out, my friends and family. I imagined every worst possible outcome, all of which, I think, involved people withdrawing their love from me or leaving me. That was the worst possible outcome of all. By the afternoon, I could think of nothing else, and my mind had collapsed in on that outcome. I was certain it would be the case.

I went to see Mr. Nichols after lunch. He somehow already knew about everything that had happened. He asked me how I was feeling, and if I was having any thoughts of self-harm.

"Yeah," I said. "As usual." I hardly took that part seriously anymore. Being suicidal was starting to feel normal to me. I got to that place quickly now, much faster than before. I knew the way. At first, I just kept pushing deeper into those dark woods, hiking through the tangled weeds and fallen trees, lost and feeling as though I had no other options. Eventually, I would find myself in that place. Every time I went back, however, the path got clearer. Strong emotions—especially shame, guilt, embarrassment and frustration—were usually the triggers that took me back there. Amy had helped me start to see that, but she left before teaching me how to change it. That wasn't her fault, of course. I learned that turnover was common in the mental health care system.

Mr. Nichols didn't have many options either. He wasn't a therapist or a doctor, so he couldn't play that role for me. Where else could he send me to fill those needs? The emergency room was pretty much the only option. So, once again, that's what he suggested. I agreed on the condition that he didn't tell anyone what I had done. Maybe sensing that the precipitating event wasn't really the issue anymore, offering me compassion despite my actions, he agreed. I didn't want anyone to know what I had done. I also didn't want anyone to know what doing it had done to me. I wasn't the victim here; the girl whom I upset was. This was all my fault, and I deserved to be punished.

I am not a good boy, Mom.

I did a bad thing.

I am a bad thing.

CHAPTER 9

I WAS ADMITTED TO THE PSYCH WARD FOR THE FIRST time in 2001, just before Christmas. I was fourteen and the youngest on the unit by a margin of decades. It wasn't anything like I had expected, but, then again, I didn't really know what to expect.

When Mr. Nichols called my mother, he asked her to come pick me up and take me to the hospital. He told her, again, about the stress, my falling grades, my hopelessness and my thoughts of suicide. He didn't tell her what had triggered me to fall back down that hole. My mom came with Gary to pick me up, and we went to the emergency room. After hours in the mostly empty waiting room, I eventually got in. I talked to a parade of what felt like a half-dozen or more people who all asked mostly the same questions as last time.

Then came the psychiatrist, Dr. Khouri. He was quiet, with an unfamiliar accent, so when he did talk, I had a hard time understanding him. He made the decision to admit me to the psych ward. All the while, my mother and Gary sat in the same small room with me. Mom, in a chair by the wall, didn't say much.

I couldn't shake the feeling that I was inconveniencing her, that I was a burden. Gary mostly stood by the door, shifted around, went on short walks and complained about how long it was taking. I think he was mostly eager to ensure that anyone who might happen to see him there, and who would listen, knew how perfect our lives were in the little yellow house in the woods.

"We buy him whatever he wants, and he's still not happy," Gary said to Dr. Khouri.

As I sat on the hospital bed in the little room, two things bothered me about what Gary had said. First, when Gary said "whatever he wants," he was usually referring to the basics—food, clothing, shelter. It had become clear that his way of expressing affection was to be a provider, the way he believed "a real man" should be. But I didn't think that providing basic needs gave anyone the right to treat people however they wanted. Second, his belief that he showered us all with riches wasn't exactly true. The primary breadwinner in the house was my mother, not him. But that didn't fit his desired narrative. Still, it wasn't his mischaracterization of our lives that bothered me most. It was the fact that he was, essentially, saying that my real problem wasn't depression and anxiety, it was ingratitude.

Dr. Khouri decided to admit me based on everything I had told him about how I was feeling. I cried, a lot. He saw that my condition had deteriorated considerably since I last came to the emergency room. I don't think it was this particular crisis that was his main consideration—it just happened to push things over the edge—but rather the emerging trend of my suicidal feelings and thoughts. Being suicidal was not how so-called normal people were expected to cope with the stresses, mistakes and disappointments of life, but that reaction was becoming normal for me. It was getting a little more ingrained each time I travelled down this path and practised this response. Resilience is a muscle, but so is self-destruction.

The stressors had been mounting in my life, and I was again feeling overwhelmed. Ever since the car accident a little over a month before, my left hip and knee had been in constant pain. It was uncomfortable to sit for longer than a few minutes. I had missed three weeks of school and was behind on all my work. I'd all but stopped eating. I'd lost ten pounds, which, on a tall, slim-framed kid like me, made me look gaunt. I'd been hearing voices in my head. They weren't the auditory hallucinations of psych-osis—at least, I don't think they were. It felt more like standing in the middle of a room where everyone was having different conversations all around me, or listening to an out-of-tune radio that was set between stations. The nurses told me that hearing voices was normal. It didn't feel normal—nothing did. I didn't even know what "normal" meant.

Dr. Khouri asked me how often I'd been having thoughts of suicide.

"All the time," I answered. "I have them every day."

If this was what it was like to be a typical teenager, I didn't want it. Gradually, I had lost the ability to ignore the thoughts. I couldn't avoid them, un-think them, escape them by the stream in the forest. I'd been circling the drain for months.

That evening, after many hours in the emergency room—waiting to be seen, waiting to be assessed, waiting for a room assignment—I was transferred to a stretcher and wheeled down to the psych ward. I didn't understand why that was necessary. "There's nothing wrong with your legs," my mother would say when I asked her to do something for me that I could have easily done for myself. The staff at the hospital didn't give me a choice. "It's procedure," the nurse said.

Unit 1C was one of three psychiatric wards in the basement of the Cape Breton Regional Hospital. It was for the acute patients, less severe and persistent cases, though it was still a secure ward like the other two. We buzzed the intercom at the locked double door and waited for one of the night shift staff to let us in. There was a fourth ward for mental health patients, but it was usually closed due to the staffing shortages that were common at the few remaining hospitals on the island. I noted that the cafeteria, and the exit should I need it, was a short distance down the dimly lit, cinder-block, pastel-painted hall—so it wasn't all bad news. Across from the cafeteria was the morgue.

We arrived at Room 1034 at around 8 p.m. My mother didn't stay long but said she would come back to visit me the next day. The nurse who got me settled introduced herself as Jane. The deep, wise creases on Jane's face were framed by a blond bob haircut. She looked a little like my sixth-grade teacher, Mrs. Peterson. I liked Mrs. Peterson, so by unconscious association I automatically liked Jane too. She was kind and welcoming. When I first arrived, she had asked me all the same questions and took all the same notes as the psychiatrist before her, the crisis worker before that, the triage nurse before that and, informally, the guidance counsellor before that. It was my first time being admitted to a psychiatric ward, but I'd already repeated myself so many times that I almost had the questions, and the answers, memorized.

"I'm always thinking about killing myself," I said to Jane.

I told her how I'd been more agitated and sensitive lately. She listened attentively, dutifully, then she searched me for contraband. Things such as cigarettes and lighters weren't allowed, which was fine since I didn't smoke. Most pointy things, like pens, were banned too. Shoes with laces were a definite no-no. They had strict rules about what, and who, was allowed on the unit, and when. She had me sign a number of papers, which she probably explained; it was all a bit of a blur that I didn't really understand, including a disclaimer absolving the hospital of any responsibility in case anything was lost or stolen. She probably could have gotten me to sign just about anything—I was a desperate fourteen-year-old kid, alone on a psych ward in the middle of the night. I wasn't exactly inundated by free will.

Nobody told me how long I'd be staying. When I asked, they were noncommittal about my commitment, ironically. "Well, that depends on how you're doing," the nurse said. "Don't worry about that now."

"Easy for you to say," I thought, "you know when you're leaving." My antidepressant dose was increased, and a hypnotic was added to help me sleep. It made my mouth taste like metal. I'd never been drunk before, but this was what I imagined being drunk felt like. I passed out, and still felt woozy for a while after I woke up.

None of the wards were designated for children or youth. I shared a room with a much older man. When I arrived at the room, he was lying on his side, cocooned by blankets in his bed by the door. He didn't move much until sometime after midnight, when he woke me up by suddenly sitting bolt upright in his bed and screaming, "We will overcome! We will overcome! We will overcome! We will overcome!"

His screams grew louder and more panicked with each incantation. I woke up with a start, confused and afraid, but my body felt too heavy to get away or even protect myself. I was panicked but locked in. Then, as suddenly as he sat up, he lay down again and went back to sleep. The room was silent again. Even medicated, I had a hard time going back to sleep. Nobody had told me it was going to be like this. "I don't belong here. I'm not like these people," I thought.

"I'm not crazy."

THE NEXT morning, Friday, one of the nurses gave me a tour of the small unit. After she left me to explore on my own, I observed my surroundings and the other patients. My experience during the night notwithstanding, I was surprised that everybody seemed so, relatively speaking, normal. There was an old lady who sat for hours in the lounge, drooling and only occasionally blinking. And there was a man with a three-day scruff who paced around in the special room with no windows or anything else. But even they didn't seem really scary.

Some of the other patients introduced themselves. The rules of social engagement are different on a psych ward. There is no need to hide, or to admit, anything. Everyone is just who they are. "What're ya in fer?" a man with no front teeth asked me in a heavy, familiar accent. "I don't know," I answered. He snorted a laugh. "Yeah, me neither." A young nurse walked by. "Hallo, gorgeous," he said with a big toothless smile. She smiled back as she rolled her eyes and shook her head. It felt affectionate, as though everyone knew him and knew he meant no harm.

Around 9 a.m., I was taken in to see the psychiatrist, Dr. Khouri, in his well-decorated office at the end of the hall. It was a nice oasis within the comparatively spartan ward. After a brief conversation, Dr. Khouri decided to change my status from involuntary to informal, and he allowed me off-unit "privileges."

"I should feel privileged," I thought, "so lucky, so grateful, to have what I have, to be allowed to go for a walk." But I didn't.

He told me he would make a referral back to Child and

Adolescent Services so I could pick up with a new social worker, since Amy no longer worked there. My previous file had been closed, however, so his referral had to wait until Monday. A conference meeting with my mother would also have to wait until Monday. That meant I was staying here for at least the weekend, regardless of my condition, because of other people's schedules.

I spent the rest of the day in my room, writing and sketching with a dull golf pencil on the back of one of the triplicate forms the nurses gave me. My mother came to see me that evening, during the very limited visiting hours. I didn't want to upset her, so we mostly made small talk about things other than how I was feeling. It was the type of hollow, wooden conversation I had grown to despise. I didn't like that she had brought Gary to the emergency room. I didn't understand how she could hate him one day and need him the next, even if I did too.

After my mom left, Jane the nurse, who was on the evening shift, came in to check on me. She noticed immediately that I wasn't happy. I had the lights off and was lying in bed, staring at the ceiling. There was no expression on my face, and I wouldn't look her in the eye. I couldn't manage much more than a whisper, so she leaned in to hear, but as she approached, my chest got tight. I felt desperate to be closer to people, but my body and mind recoiled at the proximity of others. Having both anxiety and depression was like having a brain that wouldn't let my heart get what it really needed. I craved and feared connection.

Jane remarked on how depressed I looked. After some more small talk, I started to open up a little. I told her about my difficulties at home. "Gary has kicked us out so many times," I told her. "He's just so moody and angry." We had left, and returned, probably four or five times by then.

"Why do you think that is?" she asked.

"I don't know. He thinks that I can just go outside and do some sort of work like him and get out this depression if I really wanted to."

She pressed further about my suicidal ideations. The question alone brought tears to my eyes, but she encouraged me to open up. I admitted that they were back, that they always came back.

"I just want it to stop," I told her, partly referring to my persistent feelings of sadness and stress, but partly referring to everything in my life. "I just want to be normal." I wanted to find peace. She asked me what I meant. "Well," I answered, "what do you see when you look out that window?" I nodded my head toward the reinforced glass next to me, facing out into a small brick-walled courtyard.

"It's dark," she answered. "But I think I see the courtyard, the wall, some picnic tables and the basketball hoop. That's where some of the patients go during the day and it helps them feel better."

"I see the basketball hoop and picnic tables too," I replied. "But when I look at them, I think about how I can push one of those picnic tables under the basketball hoop so I can hang myself with my shoelaces from it." I paused, crying. She was silent. "Something has to be real wrong with me to be thinking like that."

Jane comforted me as best she could, then went back to the glass-enclosed nursing station at the other end of the hall, which some of the other patients called the Fishbowl. She called the on-duty psychiatrist, who, after hearing her report, placed me on fifteen-minute checks. They made sure all the unit doors were still locked and gave me an extra dose of medication to make me sleep.

I just wanted to sleep forever.

I slept all night and woke up groggy the next morning, with the taste of metal in my mouth. Still, I did feel better. I played checkers with Harold, the big crewcut orderly who, in my imagination, had a motorcycle and played darts at the Legion where he drank cheap beer on his nights off. I liked to imagine people's stories. The psych ward was as good a place as any to let my imagination run wild. There wasn't much else to do.

My sister came to visit in the morning. As we talked, she told me, for the first time, that she and my brother, Raymond, had both gone through periods with the same kinds of feelings. I cried with her, but it helped a little to know I wasn't alone. My father came to visit for a short time over dinner. It was the most meaningful contact I'd had with him in months. My mother called, and I spoke to her on the shared phone in the hall outside my room, since we didn't have, and weren't allowed to have, phones in our rooms. She told me she couldn't come to visit that day.

"Don't get too comfortable in there," Mom said. I rolled my eyes.

She also told me that my guidance counsellor had called to see how I was doing, and to ask if he could tell my teachers where I was. He said it was important that they knew. I wasn't especially keen to tell anyone, but my mother had already given him permission without asking me and that's all he needed. She also told me that my father had told a number of people where I was. I started to feel embarrassed that suddenly everyone knew how crazy I was. Nothing gets across a small town faster than a story.

Still, I slept better that night than I had the night before, and my sleep improved for each of the next two nights. My mother and my father came to visit each day. Gary didn't, which was fine. My gradual progress continued, day by day, but it seemed to depend, at least in part, on the person who was caring for me. Each nurse or doctor who saw me seemed to have a slightly different take on my condition, having more to do with their mood than mine. The ones I saw as impatient and aloof described me the same way. The ones with whom I felt warmth and connection seemed to understand me better. I guess we tend to treat others as we ourselves feel. Caring is subjective, and projective.

After six days, I left the hospital's basement psych ward feeling more upbeat and hopeful than I had in a long time. I was discharged around noon on Tuesday. Before I left, I stood at the nursing station chatting with some of the staff while they tried to work.

"I'm looking forward to getting out of this place and never coming back," I said with a smile. Christmas was coming, after all, and I loved Christmas. The young nurse sitting at the desk looked as if she didn't hear me or wasn't paying much attention or had heard it all before.

Thirteen days later, I would be back on 1C.

CHAPTER 10

"YOU ARE NOT THE CHRIST," THE DEMON IN MY DREAM had said.

The demon was my depression. Depression disguised its voice as mine, hijacked my own thoughts and used them against me. I thought a lot about that thing that had taken up residency in my head.

I was having nightmares all the time now. My psychiatrist told me it might be a side effect of the medication. I wasn't so sure. The dreams were recurring, but in strange ways. Sometimes it would be the exact same dream night after night, but at other times I'd pick up where I left off on a previous night. The demon came back in both types of dream, and it had a memory. It remembered that it had been in my dreams before and it told me that it would be back.

THE SCHOOL bus arrived at the end of the dead-end dirt road on Monday morning, as it always did. I tried to go to school most mornings, at least on the days when I was able to drag myself out of bed. I went to my first-period class in a haze. I didn't think I was in another crisis. My mood wasn't a raging forest fire, obvious to everyone. I felt cold, detached. The feeling washed over me like a tsunami, carrying me away on a wave, a current, a riptide, my head under water, circling the drain again.

I already knew the effects of my last hospitalization had started to wear off quickly. The psych ward is nothing like the real world. It's restrictive on the inside, but at least it's honest. The more I reflected—no, *ruminated*—on my experiences, the more resentful I became. It was only partly because of the experiences them-selves. I felt bullied, abandoned and abused because I was. But the bigger part was what happened to those experiences when they entered the malfunctioning machinery of my mind. With each loop around the busy traffic circle in my head, even the most innocuous actions and events, even the most innocent or help-ful people, became corrupt, antagonistic suspects. My mind was becoming a graveyard where every thought was a body, once a person alive and happy, now dead on arrival and gradually rotting deep beneath the earth.

I fucking hate you all, Depression said to everyone I met. Depression lived in the dark recesses of my mind, but it also cre-ated more of the darkness it needed to thrive. That's how it pro-tected itself. The only sure antidote to darkness is light, so my mind learned to turn light into waste.

Every thought, feeling, action and urge came with guilt and shame, regret and rumination. I didn't know that everything wasn't always my fault, even if it occasionally was. I felt objectified because I was—I was a problem, a risk, an illness to be treated; the doctors and nurses made that clear in how they talked to me. I felt like a prisoner because I was—to procedure, to stigma, to this hijacker in my head. That's just the way things are, life is hard, it's my cross to bear. For all the people I encountered, covering a spectrum between somewhat helpful and traumatically harmful, nobody bothered to stop and tell me what was and wasn't my fault, to validate for me that this was hard but that it wouldn't be so forever. Instead, I just went on feeling so *different*, when all I really wanted was to feel the same. I wanted to feel connected.

The Christmas holiday had been a nice distraction from myself—big, distracting families have a way of doing that—but it was fading fast. It was sort of like lighting a candle in the night: sure, it was a bright spot, but it was still night. In the afterglow, when I got back to school, Emily approached me. Maybe I looked more approachable, or I more willingly noticed when people approached, when I wasn't collapsed into complete anxiety and depression. My letters apparently hadn't scared her off after all, and in the first few days back to school we started to spend a lot of time together. She invited me to join her and her friends where they hung out in the morning, in Mrs. Walsh's teaching kitchen on the first floor. Emily was friends with Mrs. Walsh's daughter, and they were allowed to use the space. It felt sort of exclusive and special.

Still, my days got worse. One morning, almost two weeks after my hospitalization, I came to school with the voice of my depression screaming in my head. Mom and Gary had been fighting. We had fled again, this time to Krista's house, where we'd been living out of our suitcases for the last two days. I slept on the couch but didn't actually do much sleeping. At school, someone called me a psycho when I walked by, and then laughed with her friends. News travels fast, especially in a place where everybody knows everybody else. I joined Emily and her friends in the kitchen. I was cranky and felt out of place. What started as nice, being invited into a new group, was turning rancid.

It was me, Emily, two of her female friends and a guy. I suddenly realized that I didn't like anyone in the room anymore, least of all myself. A few days ago this whole situation felt exclusive, but through today's lens I saw us all as social outcasts hiding in the kitchen. I responded with a negative grunt or a snide remark to every seemingly trivial point or stupid joke they made. Emily ignored me at first, until she couldn't anymore.

"You're such a pre-Madonna," the boy said to Emily, good-natured teasing. His wilful mispronunciation irritated me. Everything irritated me.

"It's prima donna," I corrected, annoyed, putting the emphasis on the proper syllables.

Maybe it was something in my tone, or it was just the last straw. Emily rolled her eyes. Either she said or I imagined her saying, "Mark, I think you should leave." I remember her saying that, I think, but my memory is wobbly. My awareness of reality was starting to falter. Everything seemed to have an aura, and that's usually what happened before a collapse. I'm not sure if I got up and left. Things faded away.

The bell rang as I arrived at Mrs. Marmulak's first-period class. I couldn't remember how I got there. I wasn't even sure if I was really there at all. The teacher knew about what I had been going through, since Mr. Nichols had told all my teachers about my last hospitalization.

The bell rang again. The period was over.

"Didn't we just get here?" I wondered.

An hour must have passed. Everyone got up and left the room. I left and lingered in the hall.

Another bell rang: the start of the next period. I found myself standing alone near the main entrance. Little clicks of stop-motion animation.

I could have left. I could have gone somewhere else. But instead, impulse pushed me toward Mrs. Walsh's teaching kitchen down the hall. It was a familiar place. I had taken classes there, I knew the space and the teacher. Cooking was one of the few things I still enjoyed. I liked the precision of it, the way every decision affected the outcome. I knocked on the door.

Mrs. Walsh answered a moment later. She gave me a curious, annoyed look. I felt like an interruption. Her appraising gaze quickly gave way to a welcoming smile. Mrs. Walsh was short, with a kind face, not unlike my big Costigan family. I felt connected to her familiarity; she radiated a motherly warmth. Some of the kids found her strict, but I liked the structure.

She invited me into the room, and I could feel the eyes of the small class on me. That's what interruptions do—they get noticed. She looked at me, waiting for me to speak. The truth is, I didn't really know what I was doing, so I blurted out the first thing that came to mind.

"I need a knife," I said. "A long, straight-edged knife."

As soon as my mouth spoke the words, seemingly independent of the rest of me, I could sense her change. Her brow furrowed, her head tilted. Her expression became a question. The demon hijacker's voice spoke.

Don't fuck this up, Mark, Depression said.

"It's someone's birthday," I lied. "We're having cake. The teacher sent me down to get a knife to cut it."

Mrs. Walsh evaluated me for a moment. I could hear my heart pounding in my ears. I felt every mechanism in my body telling me to run, to scream, to cry, to burst out and tell her that I was a hostage being held at gunpoint by my own mind.

Steady, the hijacker inside me advised. *Nervous people get squirrelly and squirrelly people get caught.* My mind began to race. *I'm fine.*

Not fine makes people uncomfortable. Not fine is not normal. People love normal. I want to be normal. If I was normal, Dad wouldn't have left. Gary would stop calling me a fag, Mom wouldn't have to work so much, the bullies would leave me alone.

People don't abandon normal.

"Shut up," I screamed inside my head. "Shut the fuck up."

Normal people don't feel so goddamn alone.

All at once, I steadied my body. I relaxed my face, regulated my breathing and met the teacher's gaze. *Look how normal I am.* My lie was just plausible enough to tip the scales from an unusual interruption back toward comfortable business-as-usual. I was just giving my pain a little help fitting into someone else's comfort zone. "I'm not lying to this person I trust," I thought. "I'm helping her to be comfortable. I'm nudging my truth a little closer to hers, even if it means distorting mine to get there." I wanted to escape, but I needed her help, so I couldn't lose her, I couldn't scare her away, I couldn't have her leave me too. We both needed me to lie, I thought. *It's only cake. Let me eat cake.*

It worked. She directed me toward the back of the room, where the big knives were kept in what looked like a repurposed apple juice can. The other people in the class faded away. I carefully moved the assortment of five or six knife options around in the can, touching their handles and inspecting their blades. I knew that I needed a straight-edged knife rather than a serrated one, because I needed the cut to be quick and clean. I don't know how I knew that, I just did. I don't even know where the cutting idea came from, it just sort of sprung up. But I did know that I didn't want to make a mess. And really, I just didn't want it to hurt. The whole point was to escape, or at least vent the pain—not add to it.

I chose the knife that I felt would do the trick. It was a standard chef's knife, about eight inches long, with a black, silver-riveted handle. I carried it by the handle, blade down. *Safety first.* I walked back toward the door. Mrs. Walsh had returned to teaching, busying herself with her classwork. I left the room, knife in hand, and shut the door behind me.

"I did it." I felt a strange rush of accomplishment. It was positive reinforcement. I was so desperate for water, I'd drink just about anything. To the left of the kitchen–classroom door was a hallway that led to a side exit, which opened into the parking lot. To the right was the long, high-ceilinged main foyer of the school. *You can't just leave, that's not how hostage situations work,* the demon inside me said. I turned right and went deeper into the school.

As soon as I got back into the foyer, I realized how it might look, me carrying around this big knife, so I diverted to a nearby bench, the one overlooking the locker pit. I was carrying my school bag by the top loop in my other hand. I rested the bag on the bench and opened the zipper. I put the knife tip-down into my bag, among my books and unfinished homework. I hiked the bag up over my shoulders and onto my back. I walked to the opposite end of the foyer and up the stairs to the second level. I saw the elevator that I had used after the car accident, when I couldn't climb the stairs on my own. That was a nice accommodation for my then very visible condition, but it needed a key. Everyone can't be accommodated so nicely. I took the next set of stairs instead.

When I reached the next floor, I walked the loop of hallway lined with classrooms. I looked through the open doors of some, thinking of the knife in my bag. I found another stairwell and walked up to the top floor. I passed a window, paused.

You could jump.

The hijacker cast a vivid image in my mind. I thought about the other students going outside and seeing my body, twisted and broken and bloody on the concrete four storeys below. The glass was reinforced by wire and the window didn't open, just like the ones in the psych ward. Middle schools and psych wards have a lot in common. So I kept going. I walked the top loop of hallways, peering into a few more classrooms as I went. It was quieter up there. I stepped inside Mrs. Ivanov's empty room and looked around for a moment. I went out and continued down the hall, past my health class, the one I was supposed to be in just then, and past the room with the pretty teacher who wore the clingy shirts.

It was a tour of all my familiar places. Maybe I wanted to see them one last time, or maybe I needed to think, or to stall. Maybe I was walking around because I wanted to give someone, anyone, one last chance to help, to ask me why I wasn't in class, to ask what was wrong. Every impulse I had came with uncertainty. I didn't trust myself. I felt as though I was walking a fine line, teetering on the windy edge of sanity, the wind on one side pushing me back, the wind from the other pushing me over. I didn't encounter anyone.

My windy impulse carried me back downstairs. In a moment of habit, a reversion to the mean, a momentary loosening of the hijacker's grip, I found myself at the guidance counsellor's office. I watched my hand knock on his door, like it didn't belong to my body. The door was partly open. Mr. Nichols looked up from something he was working on and welcomed me in. I entered and sat on the hard, steel-framed chair to my right. I set my school bag with the knife hidden inside on the floor between my feet.

"What's up?" he asked.

His face was caring, his eyes soft and tired. I trusted him. I felt my hunched shoulders collapse just a little when he asked, the first crack, one that probably only I noticed. I didn't know what to say, but he was getting used to me too, so he took the lead. My awareness was bobbing up and down like a tired swimmer on the waves of my crisis, with nothing to grab on to, struggling to stay afloat.

When I bobbed back up, I heard myself telling Mr. Nichols about my struggles that morning. I was muddled, distracted by the three-way conversation I was hearing: me, my guidance counsellor, my demonic, depressive hijacker. My thoughts were vague, general, trivial. Everything sounded so unimportant when I said it out loud. I felt embarrassed, thinking that he thought I was weak, dumb and insignificant. I imagined he thought I should be able to control this stuff by now. But I wasn't getting any better at controlling it. I was getting worse. I needed to escape because I thought it would never get better.

It will only get worse.

"I just can't do this anymore," I suddenly said to the voice in my head.

The air in the room tightened. Maybe it was just my chest.

"What do you mean?" Mr. Nichols asked. He knew.

"I can't," I said. "I just can't do it."

I reached down, opened the zipper on my bag. I grabbed the eight-inch-long, straight-edged chef's knife by the blade, softly at first. I pulled it from my bag and heard Mr. Nichols gasp. I looked up from the knife in my hand. Mr. Nichols had changed. The softness in his eyes was gone, replaced by hard fear.

He's afraid of you.

"Me too," I thought in reply.

He was still in his chair, but now his body was angled away from me. His left hand grasped the arm of his seat, his right extended in a gesture both pleading and protective. I noticed his chest rising and falling. I thought I could hear his heart pounding. *Thump thump, thump thump, thump thump.* I felt that odd mix of calm and tension, my teeth clenched, the muscles in my neck taut. My mind was blank; I was on autopilot. An occasional hard, gasping cry escaped from my lips in a little staccato burst. It felt as though the cracks were spreading, the walls listing and starting to crumble, caving in on me. The thing in my head was getting restless, grasping and groping around to keep it all together. Fall, or be felled. *Tear it all down.*

I raised the knife to my throat.

"I can't do this anymore," I said through tight lips.

I held the knife near the base of the blade, in my right hand. I felt its sharp edge across my palm. The steel tip touched my skin around the area of my right jugular vein. I felt the pulse in my neck under the light pressure of the knife. *Thump thump.* I don't want this thing inside me anymore.

Cut it out.

"Mark, please don't," Mr. Nichols's voice echoed from far away.

I closed my eyes. I felt my eyeballs roll back and my head incline back with them. I gripped the knife tighter. It cut into my hand. I took in a long breath through my nose, high into my chest.

I can't.

My right bicep flexed, the knife moved.

Mr. Nichols was on me.

He didn't have far to lunge his long legs across the small room. His fingers wrapped around my wrist. He wrenched the blade from my hand and pushed me to the concrete floor. I lost track of the knife—either it flew across the room or he wrestled it from me. I landed hard. He landed on top of me, still gripping the wrist of my empty right hand, his knee on my thigh.

Mr. Nichols held me, just for a moment. I wasn't fighting. I had no intention of hurting anyone but myself. He got up off me, released me and reached across the room to hit the intercom button on the phone on his desk. He called for the principal to come.

"Come here now," he said. "Mark Henick had a knife. He tried to kill himself in my office."

The vice-principal, Mr. O'Brien, appeared in the open door a minute later. From my vantage point on the floor I saw his wide owl eyes look down at me urgently, then at the guidance counsellor. His lips moved, but I couldn't hear him, as if my head had slipped under water. Mr. Nichols gestured toward the discarded knife, which was somehow now on his desk. After a short exchange the two men must have decided I needed to be taken back to the hospital. There may have been others in the room too, I'm not sure—my awareness was bobbing on the waves. They couldn't call emergency services because it might cause a scene, and scenes at schools had to be explained to children and their parents.

This thing inside my mind had disguised itself as part of me. My doctor said I had depression, but he didn't tell me that depression was a parasite, or a cancer, or some kind of slow and malignant growth. After a while I had a hard time distinguishing where I started and where it ended. Whenever I did have moments when I could distinguish it from myself, I hesitated to part with it. To excise a tumour of depression from my mind would be to cut out a part of who I was, I thought. Depression was an abusive lover, and I always went back. I didn't know who I was without it, because I couldn't remember a time when I was without it.

You need me.

My depression spoke to me, in images and words, in my thoughts and feelings and actions. It was taking on an identity and replacing my own. It was learning and growing, and it was convincing. It was the problem, but it also offered the solution.

Oh look, Depression whispered. *I brought something along to help you with your pain. You don't have to live this way. You don't have to live at all.*

I believed these thoughts because they were coming from inside me. I heard these voices so often that they were normal. That was the whirlpool of circular thinking in which I'd been stuck, which sucked me deeper with every cycle: the harder I tried to be normal, the less people suspected I was suffering, and the less kindness and support they offered, and the harder it got to stay normal.

Mr. Nichols got me on my feet. He put his coat over my shoulders and walked me down the stairs near his office. He escorted me down the hall, across the main entrance foyer, and we exited into the parking lot. It was cold out that day, but I was still too numb to notice. He loaded me into the front passenger seat of his little white car with some rust along the door frame. We drove off in silence.

When we got to the highway that led to the hospital, I looked through the window at the trees speeding by on the other side of the glass, I studied the ice that clung to the branches and the snow that dusted the fields. Everything was frozen. I looked down to the door handle. I thought about how I could open the door and throw myself out. An image intruded into my mind of my body as it twisted and scraped on the asphalt before finally being squished beneath the wheels of an oncoming semi. I could finish what I had started. I wouldn't even feel it. I couldn't feel anything.

But I didn't open the door. I was too tired. I couldn't lift my arms. I'd gone cold, dead, into a state of self-administered shock.

We arrived at the hospital. Mr. Nichols pulled up to the emergency room door, parked in the loading zone and walked me inside. I sat across from the nurse as he described what had happened. She looked me over, asked the usual questions, typed in some notes and sent us off to be seated in the waiting area. My mother arrived a short time later, in her nursing scrubs. She'd been at work upstairs, caring for other people's hearts. The familiar smell of latex and disinfectant lingered in the cold air around us.

She sat with me, both of us silent.

I think my mother finally understood.

I wanted to die.

PART THREE

THE WINTER

How cold I grew, how faint with fearfulness,
Ask not, Reader; I shall not waste breath
Telling what words are powerless to express;
This was not life, and yet it was not death . . .

—DANTE, INFERNO, XXXIV (22–25)

Chapter 11

I SAW ALL THE SAME PEOPLE AND ANSWERED ALL THE same questions. The hospital experience was familiar now, but the swirling underwater feeling in my mind was starting to solidify like the ice outside.

The period after Christmas had been the worst part of winter —most of winter—because there was nothing left to look forward to. I still carried a sense of anticipation and hope before the holidays, but once it was all over, it was all over.

I felt numb. This was not the disconnected feeling that had been coming from time to time when I was overwhelmed. This was new. It was more like a deadness, as though my progressively more intentional efforts to kill myself were only succeeding at killing something inside me instead. I was trying, but my maladaptive coping efforts amounted to little more than self-surgery with a dull knife. I wasn't sure yet if I preferred to feel everything or to feel nothing, because I couldn't see what was happening to me from my vantage point on the inside. It was dark under the icy cold water, and it was hard to get oriented when everything was shutting down.

Dr. Ambrose was the psychiatrist on call in the emergency room that day. I'd seen him briefly the last time I was on the unit as well, so he wasn't completely unfamiliar. He had a round face and didn't wear a tie, and he felt more approachable than other doctors, especially the other psychiatrist. After talking to me, he identified that the crisis had started brewing about three days prior, amid the recurring conflicts at home. My mother and Gary had had another screaming match, we packed our bags again, and she and I stayed at Krista's for three days. I'd lost count of the number of times we had left. A few days was typical, then we always went back.

Dr. Ambrose quickly discovered my first secret: my only regret that day was that I didn't cut my throat and bleed out all over the guidance counsellor's office floor as I died. I was still suicidal. *Considering attempts of suicide, young age, dysfunctional family background,* he wrote in his emergency assessment of me. *Admit to Unit 1C.* He ordered that I be checked every fifteen minutes.

The crisis worker, Lynn, brought me to Room 1032 that afternoon. I declined the unit orientation from Mary, the nurse. They both remembered me. Dr. Ambrose came back later that day to see how I was doing. *Little reactivity, very constricted affect,* he noted. *No spontaneity in speech, avoids eye contact, superficial rapport. Difficult to engage him in conversation.* He maintained the fifteen-minute checks and left.

He came back a third time, later that night. I liked that he checked on me. Even if I didn't always show it, the gift of his effort and time was absorbed by me, a little, through the walls I was building around my mind. When Dr. Khouri was monitoring me, I'd see him once a day, if that, for maybe ten minutes. Dr. Ambrose didn't spend much longer—I understood that there were other patients he had to care for—but he seemed more engaged and genuinely interested in me. He struck me as more active in trying to figure out how to help me, rather than simply holding me there until I either figured out how to help myself or just gave up and became compliant.

"Ninety percent of my mind says to kill myself," I told him on his third visit to me that day. "It's like I'm in a dream." My fifteen-minute checks were stepped up to one-on-one nursing for the rest of the night. From the moment I was brought to hospital this time, I was filled with darkness and expressed a firm conviction that I wanted to die. That was new too. On previous hospitalizations I had been able to swim back to the surface more easily. This time I stayed under longer.

Just before noon the next day, Dr. Khouri dropped by my room for the first time on that admission. He was in charge of the unit, but Dr. Ambrose had been covering for him while he was out. Over the course of about ten minutes, he asked me all the basic questions, then he simply nodded and left without saying goodbye. He went back to the nursing station, discontinued my one-on-one care and increased my antidepressant dose yet again. Then he referred me for transfer to the Izaak Walton Killam Hospital for Children—the IWK, as we all knew it—a five-hour drive over the causeway and across the Mainland, in Halifax. They had a child and youth mental health unit there, with nursing and medical staff specifically trained to handle the kinds of issues kids my age were dealing with. At least, that's what I was told.

That night was quiet, and I had a few visitors. One of them was Emily. While I'd been surprised before that my awkward letters hadn't scared her off, I was entirely dumbfounded now to find that neither, apparently, had my attempt to cut my own throat. Mrs. Walsh came too. She felt guilty for letting me take the knife from her classroom. I couldn't yet see how she could have done anything else, since the whole point was for me to be convincing, to be so normal that nobody would ever suspect how abnormal I really felt inside. She had reacted in that moment exactly the way the lying hijacker inside me expected her to react.

The next day, as I prepared for my transfer to Halifax, I met with the unit social worker. In a sea of people who were indifferent, more than a few who were hostile and a handful who were able to help and willing to understand, she stood out as someone who I felt understood me. Heather connected with me as someone who respected my existence and my right to be alive.

"I don't like that I can't have nail clippers," I told her. "Or my cellphone, or my pants. I can't even go to the bathroom by myself. I feel like a prisoner." The locked ward alone was enough to sentence me to that feeling. "I don't know how that's supposed to help me."

If I wasn't crazy before I got into the system, I felt they were doing everything they could to change that. I didn't understand why, in an effort to get better, I had to be treated like such a sick person. I felt as though I'd been exiled to a leper colony. I told her how it bothered me that everyone treated me differently ever since I had started struggling. Did they think I was just choosing to make everyone's life difficult? Life was hard enough as it was, without me making it harder for everyone.

"Why can't you just get over this whole 'depression' thing?" my frustrated mother asked.

"You should be able to shake these feelings off," my sister said. "You should realize how being in hospital is affecting the family." She and my father had come to visit me in the hospital earlier that day.

"You're not special," my father said to me, under the impression I was seeking attention, as though attention were the most burdensome resource to be given.

"That's why I feel like suicide is the answer," I told Heather. "Because then I'm not hurting anyone anymore. I know some-one killed themselves on this unit last week," I continued. "I can't figure out how they did it."

Heather listened carefully, allowing me to speak, then responded with surprising honesty. "It's true that people who want to end their lives will find ways to do it. Our job is to reduce that risk in hospital as much as possible, and that's one of the reasons you're here."

As for my thoughts about no longer hurting people with my troubled life, she reframed the situation. "Suicide does have an impact on family. They are left with the grief of losing a loved one, and with many unanswered questions."

"But it would be a relief for me to be dead," I said. "I'd have no more worries. I could have peace."

"Nobody knows what awaits them in death," she replied. "No one has come back to tell us how good it is. Death is final. There are no second chances."

It was a simple discussion; there was nothing revelatory about it. But it was the kind of mature, mutually respectful conversation I didn't feel anyone else had taken the time to have with me, especially not when they were taking away my shoelaces and underwear, or when they were watching me shower and use the toilet. I sensed that people preferred to medicate my experience away instead of helping me to understand it. I still didn't like the situation, but at least I respected being respected.

Heather suggested I find one staff member on each rotation with whom I could build a trusting relationship. That way I could talk to them, and they could share with the others, and I wouldn't have to repeat myself so much to so many people. I thought that was a good suggestion. In practical application, however, it turned out that not many of my health care providers seemed to like being told that I preferred to speak to someone else. I didn't like talking to the ones I didn't feel were patient and understanding with me, and they were even less patient and understanding with me for feeling and saying that.

"Nobody understands how I feel," I said to Heather. "I can't just shake this off."

"That's one of the many misconceptions people have about mental illness," she replied. "People have more understanding of physical illness than they do of mental illness. But depression is treatable and you could have a happy life. The choice you have to make is whether you are going to be an active participant in your treatment, or if you are going to shut everyone out."

That was the first time I'd thought of it that way. My illness wasn't my choice, and therefore wasn't my fault, but I could still make choices that helped in my recovery.

"But depression is hereditary," I pushed back, "so my kids might be just like me."

"It would be your choice of what kind of life your children might have," she answered. "You could make positive life choices, bringing much happiness to your family, or you could make negative choices and experience the opposite."

I might not have chosen my background or my brain, or to be victimized by people and thoughts and actions within them, but I could choose not to continue identifying as a victim of my circumstances. That idea resonated with me, and it started to burrow deep into my mind. The fact that I couldn't control everything about my life didn't mean I couldn't control anything. I left Heather's office still having depression, but with a hint of the opening lines of a new personal narrative. For the first time in a long time, I felt inspired. Maybe I wasn't powerless after all.

The next morning, I was placed in five-point restraints.

The brown leather straps were tightened, the silver buckles fastened around my ankles and wrists, the other ends secured to the stretcher. I lay there quietly, compliantly, watching. My mother stood close by. Dr. Khouri had signed a declaration of formal admission under Section 42 of the Hospitals Act—an order of involuntary admission. I was confused, because I wasn't unwilling to go.

"Why are they doing this?" I asked.

"It's just procedure," one of the anonymous nurses replied. Procedure sometimes leads to collateral damage, mundane trauma—an unintended consequence of following the rules.

It was time for my transfer, by ambulance, to the children's hospital in Halifax. The procedure for transferring a psychiatric patient, I learned, was to restrain them for the duration of the trip, regardless of their disposition. I learned to be compliant in these kinds of situations because every resistance or protest or complaint, however justified, was seen as a symptom. Opinions, objections, requests for alternatives or second opinions were all symptoms. Any hint of non-compliance was just the patient being difficult, lacking insight, seeking attention, not participating in recovery.

Unlike the pain in my hip from the car accident, which I had tried to explain objectively, my feelings were much closer to my identity. My feelings were my only truth—I *was* what I felt—so in assessing my feelings, the doctors were assessing me as a person. It was, literally, personal. A growing part of me was inclined to tell them what I thought they wanted, expected and needed to hear. If my hip is in poor condition, that's fine, but if I myself *am* a poor condition, that's bad.

When all the straps were tight and secure and everything was ready to go, the two paramedics wheeled me out of Room 1032. They came to the big double doors that opened into the corridor, the nurse released the lock, and we pushed through. We walked down the pastel-painted, cinder-block basement hallway. I was in a hospital gown and there was a blanket folded at my feet. The heavy straps on my wrists and ankles were visible for all to see.

We came to a small lobby, with the morgue doors off to the left. There were a few small groups of staff and patients milling around the entrance to the cafeteria on the right. As they wheeled me by, I had the impression every single one of them was staring at me. When we got to the sliding doors that led outside, we stopped.

"Let's get you covered up," one of the paramedics said. "It's cold out there."

Yes, it is.

She unfolded the blanket over me, and my mother helped to tuck it under my sides. We continued through the sliding doors and lined up behind the back doors of the running ambulance waiting at the curb. They lifted me inside, a few more belts and buckles were attached, and my mother climbed in behind them. A nurse from the unit came along too. She slid in close and injected me with "something to make me more comfortable."

The back doors closed, and I felt the ambulance pull into motion. I could see the sky moving, everything was moving, through the small round window in the back door. My head lolled to the left and I saw my mother. She was sitting next to me, hands between her knees, her head turned to look out the back window. Her face was still.

"I love you, Mom," I slurred.

She turned her head toward me and smiled a thin, sad smile. "I love you too, buddy," she answered.

She reached over and held my strapped-down hand, and I fell asleep.

When I woke up, we were in Halifax.

We were pulling into a busy hospital ambulance bay, and nobody seemed exactly sure where to go or what to do next. Cape Bretoners were known not to leave Cape Breton often for exactly that reason. It was disorienting to be away from home, to be so far from familiarity, and disorientation was uncomfortable. Eventually, after some discussions with on-site staff and a few phone calls, someone from unit 4 South came down to meet us. That was the mental health wing for teens.

We had to wait awhile, mostly in a hallway, until a bed became available. When it did, I was wheeled for what seemed like six city blocks through a labyrinth of identical corridors. We finally arrived at our destination, and I was settled into a bright single room overlooking a courtyard. At least I wasn't in the basement anymore. Other than that, there wasn't much change. I still felt down, still couldn't sleep on my own and still wasn't eating well. When I did eat, I felt sick, and a few times I went to the bathroom to make myself throw up.

My time at the children's hospital wasn't all bad, though. Mr. Nichols called me almost every day. There were probably plenty of people who cared about me, but he was one of the few from whom I could actually sense the care. I started having long phone calls with Emily too. I felt we were becoming friends, and I still liked her a lot. My calls with her lasted as long as the hospital staff would allow, sometimes half an hour or more, if there was nobody else waiting for the phone.

I was encouraged to attend some of the group meetings that were held in the common area, to meet some of the other kids on the unit and make productive use of my time rather than just sit around in my room. I had never experienced any groups or organized activities at the hospital in Cape Breton, where the busiest part of my day had been the ten minutes it took each day for the psychiatrist to come and tell me either that I was sicker than before and needed more medication or that I wasn't sick enough to be in hospital anymore and needed to leave. In both hospitals I worried that the more I came out of my room and socialized, the less help they would think I needed. I felt an extreme pressure to conform to my diagnosis, even if parts of it didn't quite fit. I also worried that everyone thought I was faking it. If I was, I was doing a very good job, because none of it felt fake to me.

I was curious to see what these groups and activities were all about. So I came out of my room one morning and walked the short distance down the hall to the common room in the corner. When I entered, I was greeted by another social worker. At least, I assumed he was a social worker, because he had a beard and was sitting cross-legged on the floor with a guitar. I sat off to the side and observed as a few of the other young patients came in.

I had become familiar with a couple of them. One was a tall older boy who didn't tell me much about why he was there. The other was a short, stocky girl around my age with dyed blond hair. She was in for OCD, she told me. We got to know each other a little better while making wire and bead bracelets with an occupational therapist. On a group walk through the courtyard outside the hospital, we made wild and wonderful plans for how we could break out together. I was mostly joking, imagining, but I wasn't sure she was.

The social worker got up and put his guitar away, called the group to gather around in a sloppy circle and sat in one of the big club chairs. He kicked off a discussion group. The topic was "stigma." When he first said it, I thought he had said "stigmata." Having so much exposure to Roman Catholicism, for an instant I felt both terrified and fascinated. When I was sent back to the hospital, my aunt Martha—one of Mom's oldest sisters, and my godmother—had given me a heavy set of glass rosary beads. She sent them with my mom, I assumed, because some pious people don't want to be seen descending into the netherworld in the hospital basement. I was grateful for her gift regardless. The beads were smooth, and warm, and the deep wine-red colour of dried blood. I carried them around in my pocket everywhere I went, the weight of the chain a gentle reminder. Maybe God could save me.

You are not the Christ, the demon had said in my dream.

When my wandering imagination returned, I realized that the issue of stigma was something that Heather, the social worker in Sydney, had discussed with me only a few days earlier. I did know something about that. I had told Heather about the group of girls in the school lobby.

"Don't look at him," one of the girls told the others, loud enough for me to overhear. "He's psycho."

The group discussion was interesting enough, but it didn't really help me much. I left feeling that things still weren't getting better for me, as I had expected they would, and wanted them to, and as they temporarily had done on previous hospitalizations. Since this unit specialized in children and youth, it had a teacher who came in to do general academic lessons a few times a week. Not long after my transfer, some doctor or counsellor on my treatment team—they all blended together after a while—thought it would be a good idea for me to participate in those classes too.

On Tuesday morning of my second week, I walked down the long corridor to the small rectangular room at the end. It was set up as a classroom, with three rows of long tables arranged facing a whiteboard along one wall. I sat in the front row of tables, but as far off to the side as possible, mostly because the room was too crowded and it would have been noisy and conspicuous to push through to the back. The girl with OCD was already there, sitting in the second row, in the chair directly behind me. I turned to talk to her. As class was getting started, we continued to talk.

The teacher was a short, plain man with greying hair and silver-framed glasses. He was wearing jeans and a dark plaid button-down shirt. In my imagination he drove a pickup truck and had a dog, maybe a German shepherd, like my dad. I pictured him drinking cheap coffee at a sticky diner called Sal's. I don't remember his name, but there's a good chance it was Jim. He looked like a Jim.

Jim called for our attention. The girl and I continued to talk. We were so engrossed in our conversation that we weren't aware of the transition into more focused work. Suddenly, a sharp bang echoed through the room like a gunshot. Every head snapped toward the teacher, mine especially. His right fist was clenched, knuckles down on the table in front of him, still stiff from making contact. His face was tight, lips drawn back into a snarl.

"Mark," he shouted. "Turn around and shut up."

He was right, of course. I shouldn't have been talking during class. I can see how that would have been frustrating for him. However, the sound of his voice, the surprise, his posture and his glare all combined to push the first domino. He reminded me of Gary. Something deep in me was triggered by his anger—maybe by him as a plain man in plaid whom I imagined driving a pickup, maybe by his authority, maybe by the startled reaction and intimidation I momentarily felt inside. Triggers are sticky—they drag a lot out along with them. I was still a slave to my emotions and how easily they cascaded out of control. I hated losing control, especially of myself. That's all it took. Poor little delicate flower me, couldn't handle a few mean words said loudly.

Be a man.

The self-critical voice in my head sometimes sounded an awful lot like Gary's. It didn't matter that I was a fourteen-year-old boy, because I had to be a man, suck it up, hide what I felt. Except I couldn't. The times I'd successfully handled similar situations all evaporated from my memory; anything positive from the past was discounted from the present.

As the thoughts spiralled down in my head, my heart pounded. I sat quietly for the next hour, going through the motions and writing the things we were told to write, silently spinning. Startle turned to fear, fear turned to panic, panic to crisis. After we were allowed to leave, I went back to my room. I closed the windowed door and sat on the side of my bed. I faced the window to the courtyard, my back to the door. I stared for a moment at the sky beyond the window. I longed to be on the other side of the glass. Then my eyes darted around the room and I noticed that my hands were fidgety.

A glint of something shiny caught my eye. There was a small piece of metal about the size of a thumbnail on the floor between my feet. It was a clasp from a hospital bracelet or a broken clip from some chart or another. I picked it up and felt its sharp edge with my fingertips. I touched the edge to the top of my left forearm, about halfway between my elbow and wrist. I began to scratch into the skin. The spot on my arm turned red at first, then bright red. I continued to scratch until the skin started to peel away. I had begun lightly, but the movement of my hand quickly grew forceful and furious. I was watching myself do it, but my arm was numb, so I didn't feel it when it started to bleed, as I continued to scratch. By the time I stopped,

I looked at my arm and the spot of raw, wet flesh was about an inch long.

The impulse was a test run. The trouble with my depressed mind wasn't so much the thoughts themselves but the associations between thoughts, and the stickiness of the harmful ones. Everyone gets sad or scared or angry, I understood that much. But those thoughts—and the defensive, adaptive, desperate actions that flow from them, as my first therapist Amy had explained to me when we were working together—those don't infinitely multiply and escalate in a healthier mind. Campfires and forest fires are both made of fire, but they're not the same thing. One is there because it's supposed to be, and it's contained where it's intended. The other spreads and shifts and jumps out of control, leaving a trail of destruction behind it. A campfire isn't a catastrophe, though it has all of the necessary potential to become one. Sadness is a campfire. Sadness might even be a bonfire. Depression burns down the whole forest.

I turned my arm over and moved the metal to my left wrist. I started to scratch in an even line, from one side to the other, lightly at first, then a little harder. The thin skin over the blue veins broke faster there. As it started to bleed, it hurt. It wasn't numb. The pain interrupted my escape. I realized what I was doing, and I stopped.

"What have I done?" I looked at the damage I'd caused myself. Why had that seemed like a good idea? There wasn't much blood at first, but my forearm was burning, my wrist stinging. The real pain I was experiencing seemed to snap me out of whatever trance I had frozen into. The ice had come to tame the fire, to contain the hijacker inside me. It didn't help, though. I was held hostage, and I was starting to look for ways to burn down my prison. I couldn't find any other way out, and all I knew how to do was escape.

I got up from my bed, opened the door and went out to the nursing station across the hall. I knocked, holding my injured arm behind me so they didn't see. One of the staff came out, and I asked her if I could talk to the social worker right away, I wasn't feeling well. I went back to my room, and a young social worker on the unit knocked at my door only minutes later.

I showed her what I had done, and I talked with her to trace my thoughts back from the moment they were triggered by the incident with the teacher. She agreed with me that it was inappropriate for him to say what he did in a professional setting and said she would speak to him about it. That validated me and made me feel a little better. She didn't judge me for the route I ended up taking but instead helped me to talk through how I could have handled it differently. There was almost a spirit of "Okay, we missed it this time, but we'll get it next time." It made me feel better to think of it that way. I was trying to learn that I wasn't a bad person who simply behaved badly and needed to be punished into making better choices. I was a work-in-progress, human and fallible, who happened to need my training wheels on a little longer until I learned how to drive my emotions myself. I'd fall down, but I'd get back up and try again. Whenever people helped me the way I needed, it helped. When they helped me the way they needed, regardless of my needs, it didn't. Nobody seemed to pick up on that pattern.

She and I talked a bit longer, and I agreed that my injuries should be looked at by a nurse. The social worker went to get one, and she briefed her on what had happened while the nurse disinfected and lightly dressed my cuts. At least I didn't have to repeat myself. When they were done, they left my room and I lay back in bed with a Harry Potter book. I read for hours, late into the night. When I finally dozed off to sleep, medicated, I dreamt of wizards and magic and a world anywhere other than where I was.

When I woke up the next morning, the nurse who was assigned to me that day came to check all the usual vitals as they did every day and looked at how my arm was healing. The cuts were swollen and itchy but had scabbed over. I stayed in bed to read more Harry, and about an hour later I heard a knock at my door. I looked up from my book and saw the teacher, the one who looked like a Jim, standing in the doorway.

The first thing I noticed was that he was blocking my only possible exit. I liked to know where my exits were at all times, should I ever need one.

The teacher spoke, with a growl and a sneer.

"I heard you squealed on me," he said.

CHAPTER 12

*T*HE TEACHER TOOK A STEP FORWARD.

He came into my room, without asking, uninvited. With that one small step, my inner alarm was pulled. My heart pounded hard, and my breathing turned heavy and fast. I sat straight upright in bed, book still in my hand. I felt as though every muscle and joint and organ inside me tightened simultaneously, from my knees and fists to my heart and lungs. My mind raced, but my body was frozen. He stepped forward again, into the split-leg boxing stance that Gary had taught me. Gary taught me more than I realized: to be afraid, to feel ashamed, to know my exits and to hate change.

Jim raised his right arm, his bottom three fingers and his thumb curled into a tight fist, his index finger jabbed forward like a meaty little dagger.

"You got a problem with me," he said, "then you don't squeal. You come to me. Got it?"

It sounded like a threat.

"Get out!" I screamed. "Get out of my room!"

He didn't move. He seemed to smile a little—at least in my mind he did.

"Get out!" I screamed again, with all the air in my constricted lungs, gasping hard for breath.

I raised the book in my shaking hand and hurled it at his head. He dodged to the left. I swung my legs over the side of the bed and he lunged at me. I pushed past him on the right and escaped through the door into the hallway.

Two other patients were standing nearby. A few nurses had come out of the nursing station. I felt sweat on my back and in my palms. I turned in my sock feet to the right, toward the common room. I didn't know where I was going. It was a fight-or-flight reaction: I fought, and then I took flight.

Near the end of the dead-end hall I turned, only to see the teacher stalking toward me like a bulldog.

"Stay away from me!" I screamed. "Keep him away from me!" My voice was high and raw.

Someone in plain clothes grabbed him by the arm and pulled him back. Two nurses and an orderly advanced toward me. The common room was to my right and the exit from the unit on my left. There was no safety in the common room; he could still get me there. And the unit was locked, so there was no sense in trying that door. I felt like a scared rat in the corner of a cage, about to be subjected to some cruel experiment. They were coming at me fast.

There was a bathroom in the dead-end wall. I ran in there and secured the lock, seconds before the staff could reach me. A moment later I heard them pounding on the door.

"Mark, come out," someone shouted.

The speaker in the ceiling above me beeped, then spoke in a clear, professional-sounding voice: "Attention, attention. Code white, four south, room . . ."

The voice warbled away. I leaned against the cold porcelain sink as the pounding intensified on the door, in my chest, in my head, all around me. The bathroom was small. It was a cold white, encasing me. I looked in the mirror, its thick, shatterproof surface like a piece of polished ice.

"How did you get here?" I asked the kid in the mirror.

"Mark, come out," the voice on the other side of the door said again. It was muffled now. "If you don't come out, we're going to have to take the door off."

The feeling of numbness washed over me, sound and feeling faded. I pulled the simple bandages off my wrist and arm. I ripped the scab from my forearm in one piece, taking some of the skin underneath with it. I watched it bleed, but I couldn't feel it.

I went for my wrist next. I picked at the corner of the scab first, then began to tear it away. It left a furrow deeper than the original, as the first scab did. This one stuck at a spot where it was anchored deeper. I paused for a moment. I heard the whir of a power drill outside the door as it barely pierced the fog in my mind.

I ripped the rest of the scab free and bled onto the porcelain sink. I was surprised—there was a lot more blood than I was expecting. It dripped bright red in stark contrast to the hard white surface. "There," I thought. "I feel."

My memory bobbed up and down on the waves, the bracing cold water pulling me under.

I turned and saw the door moving at a funny angle, or maybe it was me. Then it opened. I walked toward the nurses, slowly, defeated, holding my arm and crying. The light in the corridor seemed different from the light in the small white bathroom.

I felt a needle, it stung, and I stumbled.

I closed my eyes.

. . .

THREE DAYS after I locked myself in the bathroom, I was discharged.

"That was just an isolated incident," Dr. Cameron, the psychiatrist I saw two or three times, told my mother and me. It was exactly two weeks to the day after my admission. I still didn't feel any better, but I didn't want to be there anymore, either. I'd had the same conversations so many times with so many people over the last few months. I knew what they needed to hear to let me out.

On my release, I was assigned a new outpatient clinical social worker, Lisa, at Child and Adolescent Services back in Sydney, for ongoing therapy appointments. Dr. Cameron's "only note" to Lisa on what he described as my uneventful stay was that I had problems socially. "How can two people's interpretations of the same events be so different?" I thought. With my mother's help I filed a complaint with the children's hospital over the teacher. They wrote back, apologizing, and conceded that he had behaved inappropriately.

It was nearing the end of January. My school wasn't willing to take me back until they could arrange a meeting between Lisa, my mother, Mr. Nichols and the principal. One of the two school social workers who travelled among the district's fifty-plus schools was apparently going to be there as well, though I don't recall ever having met her. It seemed the only person not invited to the party was me. The purpose of the meeting was to figure out "what to do" with me. My teachers were anxious about my return.

"What should we do," one asked, "if he goes to the bathroom and doesn't come back?"

A few days after I got home, my mother and I had an appointment with Lisa. I didn't talk much, since not much had changed. I didn't connect with Lisa the way I had with Amy, my first therapist there. She remarked on the very noticeable scar on my wrist. We talked—or she talked—about how it seemed to be a frustrated response to not knowing how to deal with my emotions. I didn't disagree with that.

Lisa gave me some information on depression and, as she said, "how we get over it and how medication works." It seemed a little late to me, given how many times I'd been in hospital and how many medications I'd been on already. I took the photocopied information sheets and didn't read them. Lisa had given me everything she needed to give me, so we wrapped up early.

"We will probably begin working on the cognitive behavioural stuff in our next session," she said. She also suggested that my mother get in touch with Dr. Khouri's private practice, so I had someone to monitor my various medications. We had only one or two child psychiatrists on the island, but I'd never met them. They were very busy, I was told. I promised not to kill myself before our next appointment, and my mother and I went on our way feeling that at least there was something of a plan in place.

MY SCHOOL had their meeting about me and agreed to let me return.

On my first day back, nobody asked where I'd been for the last three weeks. I felt that everybody knew, but nobody had sent any cards or well wishes. Mr. Nichols met with me and said I should treat it like a new year, a new chance to start afresh, and not to worry about any of the work or anything else I had missed or had not done. The day went more smoothly than I expected. After the last bell Emily came to find me in the locker pit. We had grown closer over the last few weeks, mostly over the phone. I walked her home, and we talked the whole way. I felt lighter.

The next day, I again met up with Emily after school, and again walked her home. It was starting to feel like a routine already, or at least the hope of one. It was also Valentine's Day. We arrived at the bottom of the steep hill by her house and stopped near a steel barricade that blocked the way to a thin little stream that ran under the street. She said she had to get home but lingered. That was my opportunity. I opened my bag and gave her the heart-shaped box of chocolates I had stuffed in there. Then I leaned in and kissed her. She smiled, bit her lower lip, then turned and ran toward the narrow dirt path that climbed the hill to her house. My fantasy was becoming real, I thought. I felt happy. Interspersed with my identity as a mentally ill person, I was also just a kid trying my best to grow up.

On the third day, Friday, I breezed through the morning at school and almost felt normal again, whatever I thought that was supposed to feel like. At lunch, Emily found me and told me she had gotten in trouble for getting home late yesterday. Her mother had seen us from the window and had punished her with penance to repent for her behaviour. She was already gone when I went to walk her home that day, and I didn't hear from her all day Saturday either.

After church on Sunday, her mother intercepted me. She told me that Emily had been punished because of me. She referred vaguely to my recent "hard time" and suggested I stay away. "It would be best," she said. I turned and left, upset that I had screwed up one of the few good things I thought I had.

With my response to stress well-conditioned by now, the cognitive pathway from trigger to trauma opened wide, and I slid easily back down into the drain.

CHAPTER 13

I GOT HOME FROM CHURCH AND TRIED TO HANG MYSELF with an extension cord, from the railing over the basement stairs. Mom found me in progress, we saw each other's eyes, and she stopped me. She and Krista took me back to the hospital. It was my third hospitalization in three months, three weeks after I had left the children's hospital psych ward, after only three days back at school. I was admitted, wheeled back to Room 1032 and again put under Dr. Ambrose's care. This time I wanted to get out as soon as I arrived. I was sick of the hospital. It didn't help me. I was sick of myself. I couldn't help me either. My mother was less eager to have me come home, at least at first.

"I don't think he's ready to go," she said to my psychiatrist. "He needs more time."

While I was in the hospital, my mother moved out of Gary's house again. This was at least the sixth time. Nobody was aware of her plan. She packed up all of her belongings, as well as my own, and moved them to her sister Marie's house. When she told me, I was conflicted: I was mad at myself for being a little mad at her, given everything we had gone through together at Gary's. That place was hell, but I was also sick of all the change. I just wanted to settle down somewhere, anywhere, even in hell.

The next time my mom visited, she was in a better mood. She reassured me that she would be happier staying with her sister and that she might never return to Gary. I was fine with that. "As long as my mom is happy," I told my nurse later that night, "it will help me as well as her."

I was discharged the next day, after staying for four days on that admission. When I was leaving, Dr. Ambrose remarked on how my illness had continued to progress. *Mark is developing a maladaptive pattern of attention-seeking behaviour,* he noted in his summary of my care. Yeah, no kidding.

Since I was still a minor, my mother signed the paperwork consenting to my release. When I looked over her shoulder at her pretty, perfectly even signature, I noticed that it was different this time. She had changed. She wasn't a Henick or a Dalton.

She'd signed my discharge with only her maiden name: *Brenda Costigan.*

MOM AND I lived in a room in my aunt Marie's attic for almost four months.

Things settled down for me in that time. I was able to walk to school every day, since Marie lived just down the hill, and Holy Redeemer was right across the street. I liked being near there, and I continued as an altar boy even throughout my challenges. Proximity to consistency was soothing.

In the follow-up counselling sessions I had with Lisa, which were never very regular appointments, she still struggled to understand me or my life in any depth. She reintroduced the cognitive behavioural therapy idea of the connection between thoughts, feelings and actions, we talked about pleasant things I could do to change my mood, and we reviewed my various crises and discussed how I could have handled them differently. I had already been through all that with Amy a full two years earlier, and although I clearly hadn't mastered the skills, it felt as if we were back at square one. I had the impression she was doing therapy *to* me rather than *with* me.

As well, I had attracted some new bullies at school, and sometimes they waited for me outside. When I told the vice-principal that I was afraid to go outside, he looked out his window and saw a group of them waiting for me. They did that most days. I identified the ringleader, Chad, and the vice-principal called him into the office.

"He's lying," Chad said. "He's crazy anyway. He threatened to stab us."

It wasn't true, but I think I had seen that episode of *Law & Order* too, where the mentally ill person stabbed some people, so I worried that it was plausible enough. They'd also probably heard the rumours that had been floating around the school, especially the one where I had pulled a knife on the guidance counsellor. I turned to the vice-principal, and maybe he detected the pleading, desperate look in my eyes. I scratched at the scar on my wrist, as I often did when I was anxious; it seemed to itch more at those times. He almost certainly recalled seeing me lying in a heap on the guidance office floor.

The vice-principal instructed Chad, in no uncertain terms, to stay away from me or face the consequences. He seemed to know I was the victim without me needing to say any more, and I was grateful for that. Still, from a treatment perspective, I was sick of repeating the same stories, to the same people, only to be given the same pamphlets and pills but never much else. I felt stuck. Why do we keep doing something that isn't working? I still lacked the practical knowledge, applied skills and guided practice on how to actually get better. Talking about the basic concepts all over again wasn't especially helpful; I needed help *doing* them.

Lisa did, at least, eventually come to a better understanding of our home situation at Gary's. She found out that Mom and I had moved out and that we had done it quite a few times before. I think it was easier for my mom to believe there was something broken in my brain than in our home. Mom downplayed domestic issues as a factor in my struggle. "Besides," she said, "Gary's not even in the picture anymore."

"I believe there is more to it than that," Lisa said.

Even if I didn't have any new skills to cope, being out of Gary's house seemed to stabilize me. I still experienced low moods, low self-esteem, irritability and social anxiety, but they didn't trigger any major crises. I was still struggling in school, but at least I wasn't failing. I dated, and broke up with, another girl, and it hardly affected me at all. Emily started calling regularly again, and we talked at length on the phone. We finally set up a date. We met at a convenience store on Victoria Road.

She arrived dressed full-on, head-to-toe goth. I had never seen anything quite like it before. At first, I thought it was a costume. No detail was spared. From the black ribbon in her hair to the black lipstick and extra clip-on piercings, to the long black coat, all-black clothes, black fishnets and black combat boots, she was fully committed. I had no idea this was as significant a part of her life as it now appeared to be, especially considering how overtly Catholic her family seemed. I started to realize that maybe nobody's family was quite as it appeared. I couldn't help but think I was a part of some rebellion against her ultra-Catholic family, particularly her strict mother, who didn't much care for me or my "hard times."

We dated for a few weeks, then broke up. I guess it wasn't everything I had imagined it would be after all. My only reminder of the relationship was the eyebrow piercing I had gotten in order to impress her. Not all that long ago the end of a relationship would have been the trigger for a catastrophic upset, and it often was. This time, however, we broke up by phone, I cried on the double bed in the attic, my mother comforted me, and I talked about it with my therapist. Then I moved on. I didn't try to kill myself. I'm not sure if anyone else noticed how big a deal that part of it was—nobody said anything about it—but for me that was progress. Resilience, at least in part, depends as much on environment as it does on skills. We were in a stable home.

I wasn't spending as much time stuck in my own head anymore. My cousin Catherine—Marie's youngest daughter, who was a year or two older than me and enthusiastically welcomed us into her home—helped to cheer me up and took me out with her own group of friends. She was a beautiful, gregarious, popular high school student, and for the first time in my life I felt I was part of an in-crowd. It gave me a taste of what it was like to be a normal teenager—and that's all I wanted.

A few days after my fifteenth birthday, I went with Catherine and a group of her friends to a Friday night house party across town. I had never been to one and, before I started hanging out with the big kids, hadn't really drunk much either. I didn't mention that to my cousin. We all crammed into a taxi and arrived at the house. We went around to the backyard and entered through the patio door. Our clandestine approach was pointless given the thumping bass of the music and the rowdy laughter coming from every wide-open window and door. Once inside,

I sat on the couch next to two people I didn't know. Someone handed me a red plastic cup of something, so I drank it.

The night went on and more and more people arrived in a steady stream through the back door. As my cup emptied, and refilled, and emptied again, I became more talkative with the strangers. That had never happened before either. I thought everyone was becoming more fascinating by the minute, and I cared less and less what they thought about me. I got up—and stumbled a little with the unexpected verticality. I regained my balance and oozed forward. I explored the lower floor, pushing through the crowded hall into the kitchen. I found Catherine, asked her where the bathroom was, and she told me to go upstairs.

I carefully climbed the thick-carpeted stairs. At the top, from a partially closed bedroom door on the right, I heard the moans and creaks of at least two people, possibly more, having sex. I continued along the short, narrow upstairs hall and came to the bathroom a little farther up on the left. Someone was sleeping in the bathtub. He looked comfortably confused. I didn't have a chance to go; there were too many people milling in and out of the doorway to the little lavatory, not to mention bathtub boy.

Then there was an audible buzz among the crowd, a sudden change in the air. People started moving en masse past the bathroom door as though they were all parts of one organism that had just woken up. The guy in the bathtub stirred. Catherine pushed through the stream of people in the hall, into the bathroom, and grabbed me by the elbow.

"Mark, we have to go," she said. "The cops are here."

The anxiety in the air of the booze-soaked, pot-scented, hormone-laced house was gaining energy fast. As Catherine and I made our way back toward the second-floor bathroom door, a boy not much older than us raced past. Without any hesitation at all, he hauled himself up and out the open second-floor bath-room window and disappeared.

When we came back down the stairs, two police officers were standing at the back door. With no doubt the worst possible timing in the history of underage partying, a fight broke out in the middle of the living room.

The cops advanced to break it up, and Catherine and I and a pack of others dodged past and slipped out the back door. We darted across the backyard and ran between the rows of houses. We didn't stop running for at least ten minutes, pushing through bushes and vaulting over garden gnomes and escaping the motion-activated spotlights that apparently everyone in Cape Breton had affixed to the corner of their house.

When we finally stopped running, we were, somehow, still together. Some of Catherine's friends whom I hadn't seen for a while had joined in our escape as well. We walked now, winded, and laughed. When a cab finally carried us back home, Marie was waiting up for us. She wasn't mad. She checked Catherine's breath. Skeptical but apparently satisfied, she sent us both up to bed.

I crawled under the covers and immediately fell into a comfortable, normal sleep.

MY MOTHER living in her sister's attic was never intended to be a permanent arrangement.

As the months passed, Gary returned to full courtship mode. There was nowhere else we could really go, and he seemed to convince my mother that moving back in again would be a good idea. Maybe it would be different this time. We moved back to Gary's house in early June.

By mid-July, I was back in hospital.

It wasn't anything dramatic this time. I broke up with a girl whom I'd been seeing for just two weeks. I think we had only gone to a movie or the mall together and exchanged a few phone calls. Still, the passive suicidal thoughts came anyway, and I didn't trust myself to control them. I made no attempts or gestures, but I was admitted for twenty-four hours, then released. I was in a situation I'd been in before, having broken up with girls at least twice while we were out of Gary's house. I had hardly given it a second thought those times, and not much had changed in the interim, except one thing: where we were living. It was different this time.

Late one night, around eleven thirty, Gary told me to come outside with him. I listened and I followed. I was fifteen, but I still mostly did as I was told. I had experienced plenty of consequences for non-compliance, after all.

Gary walked down the long gravel driveway toward the pitch-black forest, with me about ten feet behind. The light posts at the end of the concrete walkway were set on a timer that didn't always work, and that night they were dark. It was a clear night. Usually, on clear nights out there at the end of the dead-end dirt road, so many stars blanketed the sky that it didn't even seem black. There would be millions of tiny points of light as far and deep as the eye could see. Sometimes I'd lie out there in the obsessively manicured field and lose myself in the stars. The harder I stared, the more they came alive, changing, shimmering, zipping around the sky. This time, though, I didn't even notice them. At the worst points in my depression, I'd forget the stars; I'd look only to the empty black spaces between them.

Gary turned off to the right just past the birch trees. The next visible light was the one over the door of the tool shed that sat on a concrete slab. It was a small, wooden, rectangular building, about half the size of a construction trailer, painted the dirty, dark colour of dried blood. Gary went inside and flicked on the lights. I arrived a moment later and stopped outside the door.

"Come in," he said without looking at me.

I obeyed, compliant. I stepped in and looked around at the dirty grey interior. The place smelled of gasoline and cut grass and wet fur. There was a deep workbench overflowing with tools and things to be tooled. Everything looked the same muted colour. The floor was crowded with lawn mowers, machines with buttons and switches, a wheelbarrow, steel shovels and rakes for the dirt and plastic ones for the snow.

Gary had a tool for every problem. There was almost nothing he couldn't fix. He had three or four chainsaws on the floor, all different sizes. He picked one up now, the big one, and admired it. I watched quietly. I was afraid, but I couldn't let him know that. He suddenly pulled hard on the rip cord. I jumped. He pulled once, twice—on the third try it roared to life. I tried to keep my eyes from squinting in the puff of acrid blue smoke the chainsaw released, the little motor emitting a deafening growl in the small space. He pulled the trigger twice, quick, revving the engine and spinning the chain. He looked deeply pleased at the sound, the feel of the motor.

He held the rubber grip over the top of the chainsaw in his left hand and the handle with the trigger in his right. He squeezed and held it longer the third time. The engine screamed, spewing a steady stream of blue-white exhaust. The chainsaw's steel links shrieked as they dragged fast around the arm, with teeth that could easily chew through my flesh and muscle and bone. The fear pulsed inside me.

Then he released the trigger. He looked a moment longer at the idling chainsaw, then flicked the kill switch. The engine died. The shed was silent in an instant. He lowered it gently to the dirty plank floor. I watched his hot breath rise as steam in the cold air. I was frozen, but my face was hot. My heart was pounding in my ringing ears.

"You know, Mark," he started, "you've got it pretty good here."

It was another sermon. The sermons were the stuff of legend. Maybe he wasn't going to kill me after all. Maybe he was just going to talk me to death.

As soon as I realized what was happening, I knew that what I felt wasn't going to matter. All that mattered was what was on Gary's mind. I flashed back—as I had started doing more and more when I was afraid, when I wasn't allowed to show it, when I wanted to be anywhere but where I was. It was late one evening. Gary walked over to the CD player on the grey tile counter in the kitchen outside the den that was filling the air with Hank Williams and turned down the volume. He called me out to join him. "Have a seat, Mark," he said. My shoulders fell. I always knew when one was coming. We were all well acquainted with the sermons.

They'd sometimes run two or three hours, and there was at least one a week, more depending on his mood. Each of us in turn sat at the end of the kitchen table like a hostage. Sunday night, with school the next day, we would be kept up past midnight to receive his wisdom. I never had the courage to just get up and leave the way my sister and brother did. For me, that wasn't how hostage situations worked. I felt trapped. It often seemed I was torn between obeying authority in order to fit in and avoid conflict, on the one hand, and standing up for myself and risking rejection, on the other. Compliance almost always won.

Gary sat in his chair. It was the one that stayed perpetually reserved for him at the head of the table. I never saw him sit in any of the other chairs; he'd opt to stand if his was occupied and couldn't be vacated, but that was rare. He needed that seat so he could see the side door, he said, and so that he could reach the phone when it rang. Nobody called in or got out without Gary knowing. That's where he sat and played the same five or six songs on his nylon-string acoustic guitar in the evenings. He taught me and Raymond to play our first single-string tune there, too. He played his guitar and sang "He Stopped Loving Her Today," about a man who loved his wife until he died, from his seat at the kitchen table almost every night. We knew it was about his ex-wife, Jean. She came up a lot in the sermons too.

I looked past Gary—avoiding eye contact was easier for me—to the kitchen window behind him. The window looked out over the smaller side field, to the only neighbour's house in the distance, and the only road out. Even from our distance Gary could hear if a car approached on the gravel before it got to the driveway. It was dark outside, and the nights were long. The sermons were no shorter, and they were often dark too. Popular themes for his sermons included how things used to be, ought to be or maybe never were. His was a world once simple, sunny and chivalrous. But somewhere along the way that world had faded to black, becoming sinful, resentful and twisted. Gary was an unwilling passenger in this new dark world, and it fuelled his lamentations.

I'm back in the tool shed. My mind couldn't stay away forever, try though it did.

I wished Gary would just hack me up into little pieces with one of his chainsaws and tell my mother I'd run away. I believed nobody would even suspect him, nobody would be surprised that I disappeared, nobody would miss me when I was gone.

"You've got a bed to sleep in," he said, preached. "A bus comes right to your door every morning to take you to school.

That's more than I ever had." He paused, surveying his things in the shed. "Do we ever let you go without food?" he asked.

I didn't answer. I rarely did. What would be the point?

"All this depression business," he continued, the word sounding foreign coming from his mouth. "What do you have to be depressed about?"

"Snap out of it, Mark," I thought.

"You know what happens to people who kill themselves?" Gary asked. "They go straight to Hell. That's in the Bible. Everyone who kills himself goes straight to Hell."

He went on for another forty minutes, admonishing my thoughts, the only ones I knew that helped me cope, as bad, sinful, unacceptable, wrong. I think it was his way of having a heart-to-heart conversation with me about my depression, and he didn't know how else to do it. Then we noticed a light come on back up at the house. My mother must have woken up. He released me, walking out of the shed, and I followed him back up the long driveway.

"Where were you?" Mom asked sleepily as we came in the side door.

"Me and Mark were just having a talk," Gary answered for me.

"I'm going to bed," I mumbled, already starting down the stairs.

"Okay, 'night, buddy," Mom said.

I got to my room and crawled under the comforter on my twin bed in the corner, still fully dressed. It was cold, freezing, but there was no sense in even looking at the thermostat on the wall. Gary had an uncanny ability to sense even a half-degree change, so I resisted my desire to increase the temperature. I lay there staring at the low white ceiling into the early hours of the morning, before finally falling into a restless sleep.

I woke up tired. I had the blinds drawn on the little window of my basement bedroom, but the stupid fucking sun still managed to get in. I hated it more now than ever. After moving back in with Gary, I saw my social worker, Lisa, much less often for therapy at the hospital. While our appointments weren't exceptionally helpful to begin with, at least she was someone to talk to. She suggested that Gary come to one of the sessions with my mother, finally sensing that he might have a role to play in my struggles. To my surprise, he came. Not to my surprise, he spent most of the hour talking over Lisa about how great the life he provided for us was.

"Nobody is disputing that, Gary," Lisa said more than once. Still he continued, and became more visibly upset as the meeting wore on. He spent the latter half out of his chair, standing, pacing, gesturing with powerful, wide arm movements. We all stayed seated, and Lisa watched him carefully. There was a very brief suggestion after that appointment that Children's Aid might need to be involved. My mother was strongly opposed to that idea. Then, in the following appointment, Lisa raised the issue that since I was seeing someone privately for help, I couldn't be seeing her as well.

"We can't have you seeing Dr. Khouri and coming here," she said. Mom and I were both confused as to how a clinical social worker and a psychiatrist could overlap services, since they each provided completely different parts of my care. One offered introductory cognitive therapy, while the other oversaw rudimentary prescription strategy. Besides, Lisa was the one who suggested I see Dr. Khouri to monitor my medication to begin with. Now she was saying that the strategy she had encouraged was the reason to discontinue our sessions. That felt like a cop-out to me.

That was my last appointment with the social worker.

CHAPTER 14

SEPTEMBER CAME, AND I STARTED HIGH SCHOOL FAR
away from the junior high where I felt I'd built such a reputation for myself. Riverview Rural High School was in an
upper middle-class community on the outskirts of Sydney. I
didn't want to be the psycho kid, the dumb one, the attention
seeker, the pity case anymore. I wanted to reinvent myself, and
this seemed to be a good opportunity to do so. Maybe this
could be a fresh start. I normally would have been well outside
the school's catchment area, but I was still in French immersion.
Sydney Academy, where nearly everyone else went, didn't offer
that program. Despite all the evidence to the contrary, I wasn't
big on quitting—French immersion or almost anything else. At
least, not unless it seemed hopeless.

On my first day, I met a girl in science class. I saw her as soon
as I walked in the door. She had long, straight chestnut-brown
hair that fell nearly to her tiny waist. She was lean and graceful,
and I soon found out, thanks to some strategic reconnaissance
via shared connections, that she was a ballerina. I watched to see
where she sat and, on the second day of class, arrived early to take
the seat behind her.

It was near the back. She arrived and sat in front of me, according to plan. Not according to plan were the two or three other boys who swarmed around and into the surrounding seats. They were obnoxious types, goofing around, clearly all in a bid for her attention. She laughed at them politely and seemed to be genuinely unaware of the testosterone swirling around her. I wasn't the show-off type, so I had to think of a subtler way of getting her to notice me. I poked her in the back with the eraser of my number 2 pencil.

She turned around, I smiled, she turned back. I poked her again. She just looked over her shoulder this time, with a bit of a raised eyebrow. I smiled. I poked her again, with a little playful flick of the long hair that fell in front of me. She turned around quick, her face a mixture of annoyed and intrigued. Mostly annoyed, I think. I smiled.

"Dude," she said. "Please stop that."

I obeyed, but I was only a little discouraged. The next morning when she arrived in class, I tapped her on the shoulder.

"I'm sorry about poking you yesterday," I said. "I'm Mark."

She studied me for a moment. "I'm Beckie," she said, and turned around.

About twenty minutes later, she turned back again. "Can you explain the clouds to me?" she asked.

She was talking about the lesson that day. It was on the different types of cloud formations. I was familiar with clouds, having spent so much of my time with my head in them.

"Sure," I answered, as calmly and casually as possible. "These are cumulus clouds—they're the fluffy ones you see all the time." I pointed to the chart in our textbook. She nodded. "But these ones are cumulonimbus," I said, indicating. "They're the angry ones." She looked up and smiled. "And these ones, they're cirrus clouds, those are the wispy ones. They're my favourite."

She gave me a look like she thought I was weird and laughed. She thanked me for my help, then turned back around. I smiled at the back of her head.

Over the next few weeks we continued to talk in class, and I found myself more openly expressing a quirky sense of humour, which, I think, had always been there but which I'd never really felt able to convey before. I sensed I could be myself with her. I asked one of Beckie's friends to tell me more about her. I was disappointed to learn that she was dating someone, and that they had been together a long time. Still, we continued to see each other almost every day, and we even became friends. As my feelings for her grew, she gave no sign, other than being nice to me, that she might feel the same.

By October, I was completely enamoured of her. That had become a predictable relationship arc for me, probably because I was so desperate to feel love and affection myself. I craved it, couldn't get enough of it, and this need interfered with many of my relationships. I was reminded of one of the most enduring pieces of Costigan advice: eat everything on your plate. They didn't have much food growing up, and especially with so many kids in the house they couldn't always predict whether or not they were going to go to bed hungry. As adults, many of them had concerns about their weight yet continued the habit of eating as though they didn't know where their next meal was coming from. I had started to do the same thing, but with attention instead of food.

On an otherwise uneventful trip to the mall—one of the few places for kids my age to go in Sydney—I spotted a pair of pearl earrings I thought would look beautiful on Beckie. They were small, off-white, with a gold back and a fine gold wire that looped twice around the pearl to hold it in place. I bought them for twenty-six dollars and, about a week later in science class, gave her the little red box with the earrings inside.

"I saw these and thought they'd look nice on you," I said.

She took the box and opened it. "Thanks," she said awkwardly. She was surprised and didn't seem to know what else to say.

The next morning, as I was taking out the books I needed for the next class, Beckie approached. We greeted each other, but she didn't waste any time.

"I'm sorry, but I can't keep these," she said. "I'm dating someone."

She handed the little red box back to me. I pretended it was no big deal. When the bell rang, she turned and left for class. I stayed back for a few minutes, put the box in my locker and pretended to myself that I wasn't crushed. Beckie and I stopped talking after that, and I mostly avoided her to hide my embarrassment and feelings of rejection.

Still, I didn't dissolve into crisis.

I SETTLED into high school well and enjoyed having a little more control over my schedule. Within weeks I'd met yet another new girlfriend—by rough count, my eleventh in three years. I didn't think of that as a good thing, if I thought of it at all. I certainly didn't consider myself popular or attractive, smart or athletic, or any of the things I thought girls liked in high school boys. I saw it more as my repeated failure to maintain a meaningful relationship and, later, as a desperate attempt to fill a void in myself.

Sarah was a year younger than me but seemed to act older than both of us. The bus that took me on the hour-long journey back home each day stopped at Memorial, my old school, where

I met up with her and changed buses to go the rest of the way home. She was shorter than me, with a sharp chin, shoulder-length brown hair and expressive eyebrows. She usually wore bright lipstick. It was a statement. I noticed.

We spent nearly every day together. Her parents had divorced too, so we had that in common. She lived with her mother and younger sister in a little self-contained neighbourhood of low-rent rowhouses and duplexes; such communities were known locally as "chicken coops." It was just off Brooks Street, about halfway between the house I grew up in on Lingan Road, where my sister now lived, and my Nana Marg's house at the top of the hill. I brought her up to meet my grandmother. She closely inspected Sarah's jewellery, clothing and bright makeup. From that point forward, my Nana Marg referred to her not by name but unfailingly by a question: "Is that the girl from the chicken coops?"

Our relationship became physical very quickly. She led me upstairs at her older sister's house and we discovered each other on the bathroom floor. It was my first time, and imperfect, but we worked hard to get better after that. In fact we practised nearly every day after school, before her mother got home, and most weekends. I was an introvert, not necessarily shy but still socially anxious, so I wasn't one to kiss and tell. Sarah was not as reserved, so it didn't take long for people who knew her to find out. It didn't really bother me, since I gained a certain desirable reputation among boys my age, and I didn't even have to say anything to get it.

However, not everyone was so impressed. One of them was a hulking Neanderthal named Bruce. I had never met him before, and I wasn't entirely sure who he was until later. It was late one afternoon after school, on the bus from Riverview. I had to switch buses in the parking lot at Memorial for the rest of the journey back to Gary's. Although I had started a new life at a new school, it seemed I just couldn't leave either of those places behind.

I heard his laughter first. It was too deep for a kid who was riding a school bus, but I suspected he'd probably been held back a few grades. He practically had a five o'clock shadow. And he was hard to miss: he got on at Sydney Academy and stood for the entire rest of the ride. I was sitting a few rows back, on the passenger side of the centre aisle. What started as some ribbing over the rumours he had heard of my extracurricular sexual activities quickly escalated. He loudly proclaimed his doubts about the stories to everyone around him. I wasn't arguing with him; he was only the latest in a long line of lunkheads who taught me that there was no point in responding.

"I bet he hasn't even gotten his dick wet!" he shouted with a smile. He said it to everyone on the bus except me, but nobody had asked. In fact, nobody seemed to really care, or even play along. He followed this proclamation with what sounded like a gurgle and a series of some sort of snorting sounds that, maybe, was supposed to be laughter.

I disagreed, passively at first, but I was getting annoyed. I was starting to feel a boastfulness bubble up inside me, and he seemed to sense immediately that he was getting to me. He fed off my agitation. As we came to a stop in the parking lot of the junior high, with me and the dozen or so other kids standing up to get off the bus, he made his move. He charged down the centre aisle toward me. He arrived in an instant and grabbed me. I didn't even have time to think.

He had me by the loop at the top of the school bag on my back, along with a fistful of T-shirt collar. He heaved me backwards up the aisle toward the front of the bus. It felt as though I'd gotten my clothes caught in a car door and was being dragged helplessly away. As he hauled me down over the step, I made direct eye contact with the bus driver. "Why isn't he doing anything?" I wondered, panicked, but couldn't speak.

Bruce whipped me around outside, and with a shove we were locked in the circling dance of a middle school parking lot brawl. The other kids rushed off the bus behind us, and a few who were waiting nearby ran over and crowded around in a circle. Sarah was among the crowd.

Bruce charged forward again, fist raised and cocked. I tried to dodge, but way too late. His right fist connected with my forehead so hard and fast that it felt in an instant as if my whole face was exploding. I still didn't even know who he was. I stumbled to the side, then went down like a sack of hammers. He came down with me, grabbing me by the front of my shirt, drawing his other arm back. He punched me in the head again, and then again. I saw blood in my eyes, and through the ringing in my ears I heard a woman scream in the distance.

"Hey," she said. "Hey! Stop!"

Everything was spinning. My vision was fading in and out. I saw Mrs. Walsh, my old cooking teacher, emerge from the side door of the school and then seemingly translocate to the parking lot. She shouted again, fearlessly, and charged between us. Big bad Bruce backed off at the sight of the small, fierce woman. She helped me up off the ground and hurried me away, back inside the school, her arm around my shoulder.

A minute later, I looked at myself in the big mirror in the boys' bathroom, the one down in the locker pit. There was a heavy line of blood streaking down the left side of my face, from my pierced eyebrow, staining the shoulder of my shirt. Mrs. Walsh was in there with me, standing off to my mirror-left. I felt hot and confused, and my mouth tasted wet and alkaline.

I pulled away from the sink and walked in an aimless, stumbling circle, from the mirror, to the stalls, past the urinals, the door, then back to the mirror again. I did it two or three more times. On the next round I made it past the stalls but stopped in front of the urinals and staggered. Mrs. Walsh came forward to hold my arm, but she was too late. I went down. I hit the floor hard. As I did, that's where my already choppy memory ends. When I hit the ground, I began to convulse.

I was told later that my back arched and my bladder released as the seizure swept over my body. It lasted for a few minutes, then I became still. Then another seizure started. The rounds of violent, full-body tremors continued every few minutes. When the paramedics arrived, they gave me an injection. My mom had seizures, usually once every few years, so I knew this injection was to try to stop me from biting off my tongue or choking on the foam gurgling from my throat.

The Valium seemed to have little or no effect. As the clusters of seizures continued in the ambulance, they gave me several more injections. One of the paramedics attempted to insert an airway down my throat. The muscles were contracting so hard and often that she couldn't get the tube in. She prepared me for an emergency tracheotomy in case it was needed.

When we arrived at the hospital, I was rushed through the ER and eventually to the intensive care unit. I was placed in a medically induced coma, to let my body rest. The doctor was able to properly insert the respirator tube once I was fully non-responsive. The paramedics said they had given me enough sedative to knock out a large man; they had no idea why it wasn't stabilizing a hundred-pound kid. While I was in the coma, my mother called her mother and asked her to come pray at my side.

Nana Ag arrived, saw me and told my mother to call our

priest. Father Errol came immediately to perform an anointing. The idea was that, if I should die, I would be prepared for the journey thereafter.

According to the rituals of the Church, the priest was to apply the blessed oil to my hands and head, recalling the wounds of Christ. I liked serving mass with Father Errol because of his relaxed style, but in matters of life and death the Catholic Church doesn't fool around. He would have been compelled to read the prayer exactly as it is written.

"Through this holy anointing," he was instructed to say, "may the Lord in his love and mercy help you with the grace of the Holy Spirit."

Mom and Nana Ag looked on as the doctor worked and the priest prayed.

"May the Lord, who frees you from sin, save you and raise you up."

CHAPTER 15

I WAS RELEASED FROM HOSPITAL ABOUT TWO WEEKS LATER. I made a full recovery from the concussion and subsequent seizures that I had sustained from the fist to the head, head to the asphalt, repeated a few times.

After I was disconnected from the ventilator and woken up from the coma, the neurologist ran me through every kind of test and machine I could imagine. I experienced a symphony of buzzing, whirring and clunking noises from the MRI, the whining of tuning forks on my head and the flashing of strobe lights in my eyes. They took blood from both my arms and used a long needle to tap my spine like a maple tree. The treatment team moved quickly, comprehensively, and at one point even talked of an airlift transfer for specialized treatment in Toronto. They thought there might be something wrong with my brain, rather than my behaviour, after all.

The results of the tests were largely inconclusive. There were a few wonky numbers and levels here and there, especially from the spinal tap, but nothing that added up to anything pathological. The doctors ultimately attributed the incident to my body's reaction to severe head trauma. Another contributing factor may have been my seizure threshold, which could have been lowered by the antidepressant and the antipsychotic I was taking. The latter was prescribed off-label to help me sleep when the sleeping pill was found to be causing memory loss and lethargy—not to mention the awful metal taste in my mouth.

After spending my share of time in the hospital's basement psych ward, I found things very different up on the fourth floor. It's where my mother worked, for one. It was easier for her to come and visit me, and she didn't even have to change out of her uniform first. I received Get Well Soon cards and gifts from family, friends, teachers and classmates whom I hardly even knew. That rarely happened in the basement psych ward either. Aunt Martha came this time, my godmother who had given me the heavy rosary beads. The fourth floor is closer to heaven than the basement psych ward, after all. She looked satisfied to see the beads on my nightstand, where I could reach for them when I was lonely. They let me go to the chapel here as I wished, and I didn't require "privileges" to do so.

I left the hospital feeling cared for, repaired in some way. When I got out, Sarah and I picked up our relationship right where we left off. One evening, we were having sex on her living room couch. Our clothes were in a pile on the floor. It was late, and Sarah's mother was supposed to be gone for most of the night.

Then, through the space between the drawn curtains, we saw her headlights pull into the driveway. We both bolted up from the couch. I had my shirt back on in a flash but fumbled around with my jeans. The car door closed outside, footsteps crossed the gravel toward the walkway in front of the house. Sarah was mostly dressed, but I seemed to forget how to put my pants on. I got one leg through while the other stabbed around in the air below me without art or accuracy.

A shadow passed in front of the picture window, illuminated from behind by the street lights and silhouetted through the white cotton drapes. Steps approached the door. Sarah ran to the door, secured the chain lock and the deadbolt. Keys jingled on the other side. A second later the bolt twisted free and the door opened, clunking against the chain lock.

"Sarah?" Her mother's voice. "Sarah, open the door."

"Just a minute," Sarah responded urgently, only a few feet from the door. Her hair was a mess. I had my pants on, still unbuttoned, but I couldn't find my socks. I don't know why that seemed so important. I was fixated, of all things, on finding my socks.

Her mother shouted, "Sarah, open the door!"

"Okay, I'm coming." She looked at me wide-eyed, her long, expressive eyebrows arched, then she hurried to let her mother in. She pushed the door closed, released the chain lock, and it burst open under the angry rush of her mother. She surveyed the scene, and she quickly understood.

"Where's the rubber?" she asked, her first words upon entering the house.

Sarah froze. I scanned for the nearest escape and saw my socks on the end table.

"Where's the rubber?" her mother demanded.

"There, it's over there," Sarah answered, red-faced, pointing across the room to the discarded condom.

Her mother glanced in the direction Sarah pointed, then she turned and stomped down the hallway. She stopped, opened the closet, grabbed my coat, came back with her arm stretched out toward me, her own expressive eyebrows furrowed over little balls of molten lava.

"You have ten seconds to get out of my house," she said.

I only took five. Before I scurried away, I grabbed my socks and stuffed them into my pocket. I took my coat and shoved my feet into the sneakers by the door that I was pretty sure were mine, flattening the backs like slippers.

"I'm sorry," I said as I fled, not looking back.

I jogged up the street and around the corner, my sneakers flapping beneath my heels, my coat bundled in my arms, the zipper of my pants still down. It took me about ten minutes before I realized I wasn't being chased. The mid-March night air was cool. There was still snow on the ground. It had been a long, stubborn winter. I slowed to a stop at the curb, under a street light, sweaty and panting. I finished dressing myself. I put on my coat, fixed the backs of my shoes, pulled up my zipper.

I looked around the empty streets and mostly quiet houses. It was Sunday night, and not many people were out this late. It was funny at first, or at least it could have been. Even light gets sucked down the black hole of a shame spiral. I was left with only my dangerous thoughts. "I'm so embarrassed" quickly became "I'm so ashamed." That led to "I shouldn't have done that," which jumped to "I'm such an idiot." Then the consequences began to spin: "What if I can't see her again? What if she tells everyone? What if she tells my mother?" My voice blurred with the other one in my head.

She's going to tell your mother.

That was the worst possible outcome. I may have been fifteen years old, but my mother was still the most important person in my life. For everything we'd been through, all the runs from Gary's house, even all the times I felt as though she just didn't understand me, she was still the most important person in my life.

"If Sarah's mom tells my mother, then my mother will look at me differently, maybe she won't love me like her little boy anymore, maybe she'll abandon me and then I won't have anyone. I have to escape. I can't be alone anymore. I have no other option."

You will be alone.

I circled the drain. As the walls of my perception collapsed around me, it made the world and my thoughts ever smaller and darker. I wandered the streets almost entirely dissociated. It was an otherwise normal teen drama. It probably would have gotten me a few laughs and backslaps later. It probably would have even earned a firm, approving handshake from Gary and a proud hair tousling from my dad. But I couldn't consider any of that. To me, it all seemed so catastrophic, so damning, so *bad*.

I looked up from my feet, my eyes open but my mind almost entirely closed. I didn't know where I was or how I had gotten here. I knew these streets and had known them all my life, so it was easy to walk the route on autopilot. But part of me had thought I was done with all this. Yet still, stripped down, my feet, my mind, they just knew the way on their own and they carried me away. It was too hard to feel, so I thought instead, and I thought that I didn't have any other choice. I can't say I chose to initiate the plan that had been building itself in my brain, piece by piece. It was more that, once the plan was set in motion, I was powerless to stop it.

Each run through this pattern in my mind was in one way less impulsive but in another less intentional. It didn't come out of nowhere, and I learned more with each pass, added new information and actions each time. But I also felt as if I couldn't control it. It was like driving somewhere you go every day, then one day you get there and you realize you don't remember the drive. With practice came habit; my mind figured it out and I went along for the ride, closer each time to the edge. I had become addicted to suicide. Early on, I flapped and flailed in the wind, waiting for someone to catch me. I revisited old familiar places, reached out from my isolation, practically begged for help, in my own way, or so I thought. This time, however, I was alone. Now I wanted to die alone.

The trivial triggers for my crises didn't matter much anymore. I wouldn't have been triggered so easily had there not been something to trigger in the first place. If one domino falls on its own, it's no big deal. It's the successive lining up and falling down of dominoes, a chain of cause and effect, carefully built over time and trial and error, that creates the problem. Eventually, the chain can be built to produce a pathway to a predictable effect.

I reached the familiar location on the overpass, the bridge that stretched over the old steel plant, over which we drove every day. The dominoes were falling. By the time I reached the bridge, the automation, the emotional contingency plan, the escape, was well under way. The red button had been pushed, the doors locked down, the sirens went off, and the rehearsed, designated pathway was followed. My past crises were like fire drills: an opportunity to learn. This was not a drill. My mind was on fire.

A black-and-white solution is very attractive in an emergency. Get out—that's all that mattered. The path of least resistance for me, I thought, was to die. It's all I knew. I approached the railing of the bridge. I walked along it, looked over. It was the only way out.

This place had once been so vital. The plant had provided jobs, income, security. It gave people purpose. It gave people life. But now, it had been mostly abandoned. The bones of its buildings were still there, but the walls were crumbling and collapsing in on themselves. Now it lay quiet, decaying into time, forgotten and empty inside. This place that had been so central, so full and vibrant, so useful, now stood empty and toxic. The people who once found it important had more or less moved on. Thinking that nobody understood how I felt, I connected to a place that did. It wasn't the stream in the woods anymore, purposeful and dynamic under the dappled summer light breaking through the trees above me. This time, it was a useless, exhausted old work site, lonely and spent, in the middle of a late winter night.

I was tired of hiding in plain sight. Everyone knew my story. I could tell by the way they stopped talking when I came into the room, or the sidelong glances, or the feeble attempts to instruct or moralize when we had a quiet moment together. Doctors and priests, parents and grandparents, thirty-odd aunts and uncles, a hundred or more cousins, all seemed to carry an opinion on their face. At least, that's the meaning I applied to everyone. I was the troubled kid from the broken home, the one who wasn't going to amount to anything. Like the steel plant, I was useless, contaminated, my vitality was gone, it was time to close down.

Except I still had a fire inside me. I didn't know how to harness it, to express it, but I was restless. I was certain that I wouldn't go gentle into the night. I'd sooner tear it all down.

I came to a light post at the edge of the bridge. It was tall, dull-grey steel, reaching gracefully toward the black sky, no stars, then at the last second it curved quick and round and terminated in a burst of yellowish incandescent light. I stopped there, under the light, with the post to my left. The abandoned plant property stretched out below me, the harbour beyond that, the unreachable horizon beyond that.

There were three tall wooden poles, made dark and dirty by time and fate, connected by two rusty steel X-braces across the middle. They stood holding up a web of useless metal wires, long after they didn't need to hold them anymore, obstructing my sightline to the left. I traced the slender, splintered length of the tall wooden poles down, down, down to the worn-out ground below.

This was the spot. I asked myself, in a moment, if I should stop.

"For what? To be that crazy kid?"

I wondered, briefly, if I could hang on. Even just one more day, one more minute.

"I've held on and things haven't gotten better.

"I tried. But I'm tired. Everyone else is tired of me too. I can't blame them.

"Why would I keep trying when nothing has been working?

"That's what crazy people do.

"I'm not crazy."

Mom had told me, "It's your cross to bear."

You are not the Christ.

"Be a man," Gary said, often.

"I can't."

I didn't want to just cope. I needed to hope that tomorrow could somehow be different, and clinging to that hope was what had kept me alive so long. With no one to help me hope, it too eventually flickered and died. So I was left with no choice. This was the only way.

The railing looked like a short, wide, dull-grey ladder that ran the length of the bridge. It had four tubular rungs that came up to about my chest, the top two curving inward toward the road. I climbed the rungs of the railing, using the light post to my left as a guide. The road and an occasional passing car were behind me. The metal railing was cold and speckled with light rain. I didn't worry about the danger of the climb, I was well past that. I straddled the top of the railing, sat for a moment to get my balance, then climbed back down the other side. There was a narrow edge of concrete at the bottom on the other side of the railing, about an inch or two deep. I guided myself down to it slowly, being very careful, intentional. I didn't want to slip and fall by accident. The street was mostly quiet.

The occasional car punctured me briefly with the sound of tires passing over the bridge's exposed section-connector beams that sliced the roadbed.

Thump, thump.

"You can't see me," I thought.

Nobody will even care that you're gone.

I didn't feel I had many choices in my life, but I could choose if I was alive or dead. That was my choice and nobody else's. This time I was determined not to fail the way I had so many times before, at so many things. I needed some control over my existence, I needed to feel I could do something right for a change. I needed something, anything, to be certain about. It didn't matter if I actually *had* choices. I didn't see them. My brain, my mind, my life had been hijacked.

I felt my toes reach the concrete edge, just below the last rung of the railing. My feet were bare in my worn-out runners, my socks still in my pocket. I steadied myself on the balls of my feet, nothing under my heels, facing the railing that now had the road on the other side. My right hand was still holding the light post.

I let go, and spun myself around in a half pirouette so that the railing was behind me.

My heels balanced on the inch or two of concrete; my toes hung in the midnight air. There was no room for error. I probably couldn't go back now even if I wanted to. I didn't. My arms stretched out to either side, along the cold, wet railing behind me, barely holding me there, crucified.

"May the Lord, who frees you from sin, save you and raise you up," the priest had read, from the last rites prayer. "Blessed are they who mourn, for they shall be comforted," the prayer cards in the church said, the church where our whole family had been raised. "The rain fell, and the floods came, and the winds blew and buffeted the house," the plaque at Nana Ag's said, the one that didn't mention the part about the house that collapsed.

The railing pressed against my back. I felt the rain under my fingers. I was aware of the danger, and of how unacceptable what I was about to do was.

"You should realize how being in hospital is affecting the family," my sister had said.

I finally looked down. I looked past my shoes, to the ground below. A thick carpet of dead grass and brush, light brown and tangled, covered the landing in uneven patches. A rusted chain-link fence topped with barbed wire separated the ground diagonally below me, cutting through my grandmother's backyard. Everything in her backyard was the same shade of flaking grey. Seeing my grandmother's backyard from above triggered a flood of memories, and memories of stories, the two mingling into one truth. I watched the dynamiting of the steel plant smokestacks from back there, on Nana Ag's side of the fence, where she used to prop up the laundry lines with the tall wooden poles. I thought about how I would come in, after playing back there, and eat magic soup and smell baking bread as I sat with my mother in my grandmother's kitchen. That was the kitchen where Mom had learned to be a peacemaker, to be quiet and eat her soup, to pray the rosary on her knees every Saturday night. That was all another life.

"I'll need to jump out as far as I can," I thought. "If I land on the fence, it'll hurt. And I don't want to hurt anymore. I can't fuck this up again."

Black-and-white is comforting when everything looks grey. I stood there for a while, I don't know how long, clinging lightly to the barrier behind me, listening to my depression lie to me. The gravel-voiced demon lied to me using my own mind, in my own thoughts. I looked out over the grounds of the abandoned steel plant. It seemed I'd been struggling my entire life, all fifteen years of it.

Then an interruption.

A man's voice, over my right shoulder.

"You don't look like yer doin' so good there," he said in his round Maritime accent.

I didn't answer. He sounded far away. I could sense him approach, slow, cautious, closer but not too close. He approached the railing beside me, a few feet away, beyond my fingertips and out of arm's reach. Only a trickle of things happening outside my collapsed mind were actually getting through. The whole world was on the other side of the glass, and the glass was dirty and dark.

From what I could manage to see, out of the corner of my eye, the stranger who interrupted me was wearing a light-brown jacket. I couldn't see his face as he looked out over the horizon. Because of the way I was balanced on the edge, with my arms draped over the railing behind me, if I had turned too far to look, I would have fallen. I didn't want to fall. I wanted to jump. I returned my gaze to the dark, distant skyline, dotted by the mill's dead dock cranes and the freezing Atlantic beyond them.

The stranger in the light-brown jacket talked to me. I don't remember about what. He talked to me for a while. I don't know for how long. I didn't talk back much, but I listened, at least a little. He clearly wasn't an expert at pulling kids off bridges. He wasn't particularly comforting, or deep, or intentional. He was just *there*. I didn't want another person telling me about all the things I should do, could do, but probably wouldn't do. I just wanted someone who was there. Someone real, who wasn't going to try to fix me or scold me or preach to me about all the things that were wrong with me. I wanted someone who could just be with me, maybe show me how to live.

This stranger was good at being quiet, too. Not stifled silence, but a silence I felt, the kind that gets you out of your own way and allows space for someone else. Maybe he was looking for the right words, or just didn't know what to say anymore. "That's okay," I thought. "People don't always have to have an answer for everything."

Over the course of our mostly one-sided, sparse conversation, he didn't try to tell me that everything would be okay. *How would you know?* He didn't give me any of the empty motivational platitudes. "Tomorrow's another day!" *That's the problem.* He didn't say that what I was doing was wrong, or that I was selfish, or sick, or too young to understand.

We talked about my mom, my sister, my brother, but he didn't tell me how much I would hurt them if I died. Even if he had, I wouldn't have believed him. "Everyone will be better off without me." I thought I was doing them all a favour, saving them the trouble of me.

Instead, the stranger in the light-brown jacket asked me about my life. He asked about my interests, my passions, the people and places and things that I cared about. He asked me to tell him about myself with what I felt was a genuine interest in getting to know my story. It didn't seem to bother him that I didn't answer much, even if I still heard him. I could hear him a bit more with each minute that ticked by. It was comforting to have someone stand with me. The little I said, he heard. He saw me. He didn't leave. Maybe it's because he stayed that, for those few minutes, I did too.

My awareness, my memories, bob up and down on the waves, pulling me under the icy cold waves. I didn't see or hear the police arrive, they just kind of emerged. I saw the flashing lights behind me from the corner of my eye and I was surprised. I looked to my right, to my left, beyond my fingertips, and saw that the police had set up a wide restricted perimeter around me. They had parked their police cars across the lanes of the bridge and had set up yellow wooden sawhorse barricades in both directions. There were two police cars on either side. I didn't even know when it happened or how long they had been there.

Time moved more slowly when I was in the collapsed house in my head. It gave me time to think and rest. Whenever I emerged, everything felt as if it was moving too fast for me. When I noticed that the police had arrived, everything started moving very fast.

Crowds had gathered on either side of the barricades. In small towns, it's a common pastime to listen to the police scanner to see if there's any action worth checking out. The bystanders were a good distance away, but I could still see their faces under the yellow street lights, highlighted by the occasional red and blue from police cars. I remember the people on the sidelines better than the man right next to me. That was often the case.

Maybe it was a matter of shifting focus. Just like how, sometimes, I'd forget the stars and instead look only at the empty black spaces between them.

I could hear chatter, a low static. It may have been the out-of-tune radio that occasionally flared up in my mind, many people using many words to say very little. I could hear a small group of young men, three or four of them, laughing from the perimeter barricade to my right. One of them called to me from the sidelines.

"Jump," he said with a laugh. "Jump, you coward!" His friends laughed too.

"That's all I am. A spectacle, an object, a temporary distraction. Okay, that's enough," I thought. "I give up."

"*I tried*," I cried aloud. "*I tried, I tried, I tried.*"

Tear it all down.

When I got the help I needed, I got better. When I didn't, I got worse. Attempting to telegraph what I needed without the right words had proven futile. I felt as though I had tried, and failed, to bridge the gaping chasm that continued to grow inside me, as who I saw myself to be splintered and split away from who I sensed others saw. When the stranger in the light-brown jacket stood at my back and connected with the version of myself inside my head, on the other side of the chasm, it helped. When the stranger on the sidelines shouted to me, at me, objectified me, I gave up. The autopilot trigger was re-engaged. Triggers can be trivial, tiny vibrations of words, for one already teetering on the edge.

I suddenly saw only black. I closed my eyes.

I drew a long breath of cold, wet air. It tasted a mixture of freshness and must.

I felt my arms rise from the railing and float to the starless night sky.

May the Lord, who frees you from sin, save you and raise you up.

I hear my heart thump.

My weight shifts forward. I become weightless.

I'm falling.

PART FOUR

THE SPRING

A Light exists in Spring
Not present on the Year
At any other period—
When March is scarcely here

—EMILY DICKINSON, "A LIGHT EXISTS IN SPRING"

CHAPTER 16

I FEEL SOMEONE.

A split second of heat from his body.

An arm reached around my chest.

It came from the right side and squeezed tight. My eyes opened, I looked down. I saw the sleeve of the stranger's arm between me and the ground. The man in the light-brown jacket had moved fast, reached out and grabbed me. His arm was wrapped around my chest, my heart thumping beneath it. He surely must have felt my heart. He held me in suspended animation for a moment. Then he pulled me back, hard, and my feet came off the edge. I felt a tugging at my back, a hand grabbing me. I wasn't afraid. My fear had frozen.

Every muscle in my body went limp. I dangled over the side of the bridge.

I was dragged backwards over the railing. I don't remember that part. I remember the stranger's arm. I remember the upward thrust and my feet losing contact with the edge, but the rest has vanished. A short flicker returns of me lying on a stretcher in the back of the ambulance, then it's gone again. My next memory is waking up in the hospital, the place where everyone knew my name.

Apparently, I was more or less lucid in the period between being saved by that stranger and waking up in the hospital, even though I don't remember any of it. I answered all the same questions from all the same people as I had for every other hospitalization. I tried to explain to all of them why I did it. The only explanation I could come up with: it seemed like a good idea at the time.

I know that sounds too casual for what I had tried to do, but what else could I say? I had a million metaphors for my feelings, but they were all imperfect at best. I didn't have words for feelings. Putting thoughts to emotions was like tasting colours or smelling sound. Besides, it really did appear to be a good option, since all my other options had seemingly been burnt to the ground. I believed that I needed to die. It wasn't true, but that didn't matter. It was real for me, and my reality was the only one I knew.

I told the doctors and nurses that it was just a stupid mistake. I told them that I wasn't suicidal, even though I had climbed over the railing of a bridge, alone, late at night. The point of what I was doing wasn't to end up being admitted to the hospital yet again. That hadn't helped much in the past. The point was to die. And the point of dying was to escape a life that I didn't think I could live anymore, not as it was.

I was admitted back to 1C for about a day. In addition to my antidepressant, the same sleeping pill that had caused problems for me in the past was restarted, a new antipsychotic was prescribed, they gave me a benzodiazepine for the past seizures and another benzodiazepine for my anxiety. I took them all, as directed. I didn't want to be labelled as non-compliant. I was still tired and defeated, so compliance came pretty easily. I just wanted to get out.

When I was discharged, I left by myself. For my discharge plan, I was told to call Dr. Khouri and make a follow-up appointment. There was no referral for counselling, community support or any other services this time. It seemed that the more times I came to the hospital for help, the less help I got. It's not as if there were a lot of staff, and there were only a handful of frequent flyers like me, so we all got to know each other. We were like a small community unto ourselves, even within a small town. That came with a comfortable familiarity, but also the deadened sleepwalk of habit. When you get used to the people you know in a small community, however that community arises, you never expect change. You don't expect people to get better, to break free, to suddenly become something other than what they are. Habits are efficient, but they emit a pollution of rigid expectations. Habits don't change. I felt like the boy who habitually cried wolf. I wanted to change.

The most helpful person I encountered on this hospitalization was the receptionist in the main lobby. She called me a taxi. I left the hospital that day feeling more restless than ever. Still, something was different. I couldn't quite put my finger on what it was. As I exited through the revolving door, I noticed the warmth of the sun on my face.

I was discharged from the psychiatric ward at the Cape Breton Regional Hospital for the last time on March 20, 2003.

It was the first day of spring.

THIS ISN'T a redemption song.

I continued to struggle with regulating my emotions. I still often felt anxious and depressed. Relationships were still challenging, especially with Gary. I still had some seizures, and my mother still had them too. It wasn't as if everything suddenly changed for me overnight. Spring sprouts slowly.

"I didn't see this coming," Mom had said about my illness, on my very first visit to hospital. I had the same feeling about my recovery on my last. I didn't even realize that it had begun—and I don't think anybody else did either—until much later.

Although I didn't die under the overpass that night, something in me did. My normally pathological focus zoomed in on a different image. It was new information, a new experience that caused just one degree of revelation, one small inflection, and it was almost imperceptible at first. The image was of the two strangers whom I heard on the bridge that night.

The stranger in the light-brown jacket chose to see me, stand by me, talking and getting to know me, as though it didn't even matter that I was doing something so dangerous, so scary, so *crazy*.

The other stranger was the one who stood on the sidelines, who saw me as a spectacle, as an object without humanity that existed only for his entertainment, who judged what I was doing as cowardly from the safety of his group of accomplices.

Those two strangers—I couldn't let them go. Especially the stranger in the light-brown jacket, the one who grabbed me and wouldn't let me go over the edge. The other guy didn't seem to care, as he shouted to me from the sidelines. How can two people, watching the exact same experience, have such different responses? So I wondered: how can I experience the same world but respond differently? I didn't know how, but I wanted to start by doing for others what the stranger in the light-brown jacket did for me. I wanted to notice the vulnerability of others, to create space for them, to reach out.

I didn't know how, but that didn't deter me this time. Uncertainty didn't scare me as much as I thought it would. In fact, I realized that uncertainty was the key. If I was going to recover and help others, I was going to have to get used to the uncomfortable fear of not knowing what might happen next, if I spoke my mind and followed my heart regardless of what people expected.

My recovery got off to a rocky start, so I didn't really know it had started at all. Recovery is an average, not an absolute. For me, it evolved and changed in unexpected ways. I still had the impulse to escape, but now it was to get away from the life that had become an unhelpful normal for me, in Cape Breton, at Gary's house, and in my own head. There were still fights at home, and we still left a few times. I had at least three more seizures. One of those ended my attempted runaway from Cape Breton. After yet another breakup with a short-term girlfriend, on impulse I hitch-hiked to Halifax, where my brother was then living. I was found lying on the side of the highway, unconscious and convulsing, around ten thirty at night, four hundred kilometres from Sydney.

One of my doctors eventually told me that he thought I was faking the seizures. He took a passing glance at my mental health history, leafing through the distinctively coloured psych charts in my medical records. Another doctor told that one, in a strongly written letter, that I couldn't possibly have influenced my own levels of certain markers in my blood and spinal fluid. The first doctor, rather than back down, suggested that those tests were often wrong. I was left still feeling like a fraud whom nobody believed or took seriously, health care providers least of all. I didn't know what the truth was, but after the antidepressant in my medication cocktail was switched from paroxetine to some-thing else, the seizures stopped.

My mood and impulse control started to improve after the medication change too. As eager as those who treated me were to highlight my symptoms and setbacks, remarkably few seemed to notice and celebrate my little victories. I did, if for no other reason than to push back, to counter their caricature of me, however much I contributed to that caricature myself with my actions. My identity had become exactly what I feared most. I felt I had been categorized and dismissed as a crazy person. I didn't want to be a so-called crazy person, I just wanted to be a person who happened to be living with a mental illness. I didn't want to be defined by my worst moments, I wanted to define myself. I was starting to realize that who I am is my choice, and nobody can take that away from me.

In some ways it was my new-found sense of teenage rebellion that helped me to break free from the identity whirlpool I had been stuck in for so long. This shift in my identity, just in time, combined with a few other factors: the saviour-stranger on the bridge, the medication change, the fact that everyone who listened to the police scanner probably knew by now about my not so secret suicidality anyway. A secret doesn't stay a secret in a small town forever. It all worked together to initiate the early days of reversing my pattern, of triggering an upward spiral of recovery.

I finished out the school year. As June approached, I was accepted into a French-language student exchange program in Quebec. I'd never been away from home before—wherever my home happened to be—for any significant length of time. I jumped at the opportunity to escape the island where I still felt trapped.

I lived for six weeks in a small, almost exclusively French-speaking town in rural Quebec. I stayed with a very normal little upper middle-class family in their tidy two-storey, three-bedroom house with a backyard. I was assigned to work at a marina on the nearby lake, where I spent hours watching the waves kiss the shore, pull back and return in an endless cycle.

Francine, my host mother, was warm and funny, and we liked

each other immediately. She took me on as almost a special project, introducing me to her friends and neighbours as *mon petit anglo*, her little anglophone. Every evening we sat around the kitchen table and had dinner like a family, something that we did at Nana Ag's house but only occasionally at home.

In the living room on weekends she played traditional Québécois music and tried to teach me how to waltz. Her efforts were in vain, but neither of us cared because it was so much fun. Some evenings we set up a game of croquet in the backyard and played a few rounds as the sun set, then went inside to a home-cooked family dinner. It was a life that I had heard about but had never experienced. It was all so wonderfully normal. At the end of the six weeks, it was painful to leave. I hadn't spent all that long with my substitute family, but we had built a deep connection. It served as something of a bandage, allowing some long-open wounds to start to heal, and it gave me hope for a world outside my own present existence.

I returned to Cape Breton feeling more independent. I had taken a risk, I had broken free, at least for a few weeks, from the path I'd felt trapped on, and I saw it through. I somehow felt freer knowing that there could be a life beyond what I currently had. I had continued dating Sarah after the bridge incident, though we never really talked about what happened that night. We talked on the phone a lot while I was living in Quebec, but something had changed in that relationship too. Early into my trip, one of her friends told me online that she had been spending a lot of time with Bruce, the boy who had acquainted my head with the parking lot asphalt.

A few days after I got back to Cape Breton, I asked my mother to drive Sarah and me to the boardwalk that lined the downtown shore of the Sydney harbour. She stopped her grey

Malibu in the gravel parking lot of the yacht club. It didn't have
the impressive fifty-foot vessels that I'd spent my summer tending
to at the marina in Quebec. It was quiet.

We got out, and I poked my head back in the passenger side
window. I asked Mom not to go far, that we wouldn't be too long.
She didn't ask any questions, simply nodded in agreement. Sarah
and I walked down the hill to the harbour and along the water in
the early afternoon sun. We came to a bench where I suggested
we sit down. We did, and I shifted uncomfortably.

"We have to talk," I started.

"Are you breaking up with me?" she asked immediately, her
expressive eyebrows in a worried arch, her voice high and tight.

"Yes," I said.

I wasn't nervous, which was a welcome change. I felt bad
about making her feel bad, but I wasn't tied up in her emotions.
It was weird to not be so focused on my own feelings that I
could actually see those of someone else. It helped that I felt I
was standing up for myself, and that I was confident I was doing
what was right for me.

"Is there someone else?" she asked. I remember thinking that
it almost sounded scripted, as though that's what you're supposed
to ask when you're being broken up with.

"No," I answered truthfully. "This just isn't working anymore."

We sat in silence for a while, as she cried and I didn't. Not
because I couldn't, or wouldn't, but simply because I wasn't sad.
After about ten minutes, I suggested we leave. We walked back
up to the gravel parking lot, where my mother was waiting in
the car. I got in the front and Sarah got in the back. She continued to cry quietly, and I saw my mother glance in the rear-
view mirror.

Nobody spoke for the entire drive back. When we pulled up

outside her house in the chicken coops, Sarah opened the door quickly and hopped out.

"Goodbye," I said as she left.

"Bye," I heard her say, muffled through the sleeve of her oversized navy-blue sweater.

As we pulled away, I saw her mother come to the door and glare at me. I felt a moment of fear, but I didn't get caught up in the thought this time. Something had changed. Maybe it really would be different this time.

We pulled away and drove around the corner, out of sight. I could see my Nana Marg's house just up the hill and my dad's garage with its unmistakable backward N painted on the roof. He couldn't see the mistake when he was standing on the roof with the paint roller, twenty years ago. He was too close. It was faded yellow now. A lot had happened since then. He never bothered to fix it. Change is hard. Besides, difference draws attention.

"You okay, buddy?" Mom asked, snapping me back to the moment.

I thought about her question. "Yeah, Ma," I said. "I'm okay."

For once, I actually meant it.

I STARTED grade eleven in September. One morning, out of nowhere, I was walking toward the tunnel to the annex and I felt a tug at my backpack. I turned, and it was Beckie. It was odd that she just randomly came up and started talking to me in the hallway, since she had never done that before. We hadn't spoken in months.

"Hi," she said, smiling. She seemed to be bouncing.

"Hi," I answered.

"Are you going to your locker?"

"Yeah," I said. I didn't understand what the hell was happening.

"Can I walk with you?" she asked, still bouncing.

"Sure."

We went through the tunnel side by side, talking about unimportant things like what classes we were taking that semester and how we spent our summer.

"I broke up with my boyfriend," she said.

Her disclosure was unprompted—we weren't even talking about relationships. She was curiously cheerful. Still, just as suddenly, my heart jumped in my chest and all the tucked-away year-old feelings from before I thought I had lost my chance with her came rushing back. I played it cool.

"Oh, I'm sorry," I lied.

The next morning, I was on the bus, on the new route I took to school since the incident with Bruce in the parking lot. In order to avoid an assault charge, he had gone through a restorative justice program in which he had to apologize to me and do community service. He also had to pay me about a hundred dollars for the eyebrow ring that got ripped out in our fight. He was instructed to have no contact with me but sent me a series of instant messages on MSN Messenger that summer regardless. He appeared to have a desperate need to tell me that Sarah wasn't a virgin when we had started dating, that he had had sex with her already by that point, and that they had started dating after I broke up with her. I think he was trying to make me jealous. I don't know why that mattered to him, because it didn't really matter to me anymore, not the way it did when he dragged me off the bus. I guess I had moved on.

That morning, I happened to find out that the new bus route was Beckie's route too. She got on at her stop, saw me sitting by the window about two-thirds of the way back and sat down beside me. She was bubbly and talkative, and I decided to find it refreshing. She began sitting with me almost every morning after that. She brightened the start of my day.

She got on the bus just outside a coffee shop and always had a hot chocolate in hand. One morning, almost as soon as she sat down next to me, the brown plastic lid popped from the paper cup and the very hot hot chocolate spilled over my left hand and the left arm of the white-and-blue coat I was wearing. It was the same coat I had been wearing when I stood on the edge of the overpass six months earlier. I don't think she knew about any of that. She lived in a different part of town, and our families didn't exactly run in the same circles. She was from a totally different world than me—even though she never acted that way. Even small towns have their own internal divisions and order. That explained why the Henicks and the Costigans never really crossed paths much, and why virtually nobody talked to me about the incident on the bridge even if they knew. We all slotted things into neat little compartments, and that kept things normal. Small-town culture is a fragile balance, fiercely guarded.

Beckie and I started to get to know each other. Each day after arriving at the school, we continued to talk. I learned that she was funny, and smart, and self-deprecating about her own naïveté. I found out that she was the oldest of five, and that she sometimes sang the wrong words to pop songs, but her voice was sweet and pretty. I learned that she signed her name "Beckie" with a little heart over the *i*, but she preferred Rebekah.

As Christmas approached, I asked her one day if she could help me with some gift shopping. "I need to get something for my mom and my sister," I said. "I could use a girl's opinion."

She met me at the mall that Wednesday evening. She was so committed to helping me find gifts for my mother and sister that were personal and meaningful that she didn't seem to realize the whole thing was a sham—I just wanted to spend time with her. I was too afraid of being rejected again to ask her out on a date, so I set up a fake date instead. We stayed at the mall for hours. It seemed to work, because the next day she invited me to her house to visit. I agreed, and it was later that night that I summoned up the courage to hold her hand as we sat on the couch watching television. She didn't pull away. I confessed to her how I felt, though I suspected she knew. My excuse for the earrings last year was that I just saw them and thought of her, but the real reason was probably obvious. I asked her to be my girlfriend. By the end of our first date, I was in love.

Over the next few weeks and months, Rebekah and I were practically inseparable. If I wasn't visiting her house, or she visiting me at Gary's, we were talking by phone or email. As our relationship evolved, so too did my openness about my not so distant past life. I had a conversation with Rebekah in which I told her a lot of what I had been through. It didn't seem to scare her off the way I thought it might. In fact, it didn't seem to bother her at all; she was supportive, and she didn't leave. I trusted her with something personal and vulnerable, and it didn't blow up in my face this time. Not much had changed with Gary, but at least having a safe person to spend time with helped offset the loneliness and isolation I had been feeling.

This new sense of security played a major part in encouraging me to open up in a bigger way. To start with, I got involved with the high school newspaper. I'm not sure how I found out about it—probably from one of the principal's morning announcements over the PA system about an upcoming meeting of the newspaper committee. I wrote a short article about some of my struggles, my journey through various treatment efforts and how the stigma sometimes felt worse than the symptoms themselves.

I was surprised by how well-received the article was among my peers. Rather than isolating me, my openness soon had people coming up to me in the halls and sharing with me about their own struggles. It didn't seem to matter if they were hockey players, cheerleaders, band members or kids who stood around in the smoking section outside even in the worst winter storms—they all had a story to tell, and they all had something in common. They wanted to tell me because I had opened the door, and many of them had never told anybody else.

I realized that many of us were suffering in silence, yet it was a silence we ourselves were creating. We had an ironic cycle in common: we were lonely because we were silent, we were silent because we were vulnerable, and we were vulnerable because we were lonely. Since the silence was one of the worst parts for me, I didn't want to continue being part of the problem. Soon after that article was published, I wanted to speak more openly about my mental health issues. What if all the silent people could hear each other? Maybe they would realize they weren't alone. Nothing excited me more than having something to be passionate about. I might really be able to help people. I didn't know how to do that at first, but now maybe I could reframe what had previously been my symptoms into more valuable skills. Maybe I could take all my mistakes, all the moments in which I had tried to tear myself down, and use that as material to build others up and do good. Maybe my struggle could be my strength.

I started talking more openly about my struggles and continued to write short pieces for the school newspaper. Eventually, I approached my high school's administration for help in raising awareness about mental health and suicide. That's when I encountered my first real institutional barrier to breaking down stigma.

"We can't let you talk about things like suicide here," the vice-principal told me. "It might give people the idea to go out and do it, and we want to avoid that."

That response didn't sit right with me. As I thought back over my own experience, I couldn't identify any point at which I "got the idea" to go out and kill myself. Intuitively, that's just not how it works, but I couldn't expect someone who hadn't attempted suicide to understand that. Even if you have a best friend or loved one who has attempted or even died by suicide, you still don't know what it's like to be in that person's head at that moment. My feelings had developed slowly, iteratively, following a long path toward suicide. I figured out how to kill myself because I thought I needed to, because it seemed like my only option. I learned that I was wrong. Learning to be wrong, to be imperfect, to embrace my fall, had saved my life. It was a realization that might help others too.

Nobody gave me the idea to kill myself. Lots of people gave me the idea not to tell anyone about it. I didn't want to be part of the silence that almost killed me.

I knew there wasn't going to be much point in arguing with the administration. I was just a kid, and a kid with a mental illness at that, so they weren't likely to change their opinion. They had all the power and I had none. I didn't like that idea either. So I decided to respond in a way they couldn't prevent: in public. As I began to research the question of how suicide happens—by talking to professionals, reading whatever I could get my hands on and remembering the counselling and group conversations I'd had on mental health over the years—my discomfort with the principal's response was validated.

There are many factors that contribute to why someone thinks they need to die, but someone else giving them the idea, as though they have never thought about it themselves, isn't one of them. I read about suicide contagion and how sometimes suicide can spread, especially after a widely reported celebrity suicide. I read endlessly about the death of Nirvana front man Kurt Cobain, since he was often cited in this discussion. It became clear to me that talking about suicide wasn't the problem. Rather, it was how that talking was done, the context around it and the feelings of either shame or radical acceptance with which it was presented. People were thinking about suicide anyway, but they had nowhere to turn and felt they couldn't talk to anybody. That made a lot more sense to me, since that's exactly how I had felt.

Having become as well-informed as possible, I compiled all my research into an opinion article for our local newspaper, the *Cape Breton Post*. It was published the next day. In the article, I openly disclosed my challenges, both the personal ones and my difficulties getting help. I called on others to open up about their own experiences. I think I likened my high school administration to Communist Russia for stifling my free speech. What can I say? I was at an age of rebellion, embarking on a crusade, and words had become my weapons of choice. The article was read widely in my hometown, attracting the attention of the largest regional newscast. They sent a camera later that day to interview me at Gary's place when he wasn't home, and to my school to interview the principal.

The television reports sparked a conversation in my community that I wished I'd heard throughout my childhood. People were suddenly talking about mental health and were doing it in more public ways. I began to notice more articles in the paper on the topic—some of which were written by me—and people would approach me to talk about it almost every single day. This led me to start a small charity to raise awareness and funds for mental health, focused primarily on music and the arts, and I was astounded by the response the initiative received.

As happy as I was to believe I was making a difference in something bigger than myself, my new initiatives were making a difference in me too. It felt good to be open. I liked the sense of being useful. Even when people pushed back, or disagreed, or weren't as passionate about these issues as me—and there were lots of those people—suddenly I found myself reframing those challenges as obstacles to be overcome rather than barriers holding me back.

I returned to Quebec that summer, this time for a study trip. I'd been accepted as one of only a few students to complete college-level French credits before entering twelfth grade. This was the first time I thought I might actually be able to go to college. I had assumed that wouldn't be an option for me, given my grades, my past challenges, the fact that it defied expectations of me. I continued to nurture my budding entrepreneurial spirit that summer in Quebec, organizing a few very well-attended events for the other students during my stay that earned me some unfamiliar popularity. Academically, I was near the top of my class, and when I returned to high school for my graduating year, for once, I actually felt prepared. As the positive reinforcement continued to build and layer, it showed me that maybe I could actually make something of my passion. I announced my plan to my sister.

"You don't actually think you're going to leave here, do you?" my sister asked.

She didn't say it out of malice. Most of the time we are who we're expected to be. I didn't want to be what I was expected to be anymore.

Ever since my mental health started to decline, and I was discovered to be thinking about suicide at twelve years old, I had barely passed my classes. My marks improved dramatically in my graduating year, after the trip to Quebec. My dream school was Princeton University—I was starting to dream big. Realistically, that was out of reach, but I wasn't deterred from finding something else. I was beginning to consider setbacks as pivots to something else. My high school guidance counsellor was also practical and helpful in advising me to consider my options.

In the end, I applied to only one school. Rebekah applied there too. It was a small, historically Catholic liberal arts university in New Brunswick, about a seven-hour drive from Cape Breton— far enough away to gain some independence, but not so far as to never be able to see my family if I needed to. I received my acceptance letter in the spring, and Rebekah got hers shortly thereafter. At our high school graduation, my mother was just happy to get the red tassel from my hat so she could put it with Krista's green one and Raymond's blue one in her memory box at home.

The summer seemed to go by as quickly as the rest of the year had. Time moved a lot faster when I spent more of my days outside myself rather than confined inside my own mind. At the end of August, we loaded up the ten-year-old Hyundai that my father had bought me for five hundred dollars when I got my licence. It was originally red, but he painted it silver for me. The insides of the doors were still the original colour, and it reminded me of how the insides of the doors were still blue in our holey old red-painted Pony.

When we finally arrived, hours later, at the residence building where I would start my new, independent life, my mother helped me move the last of my things. She hugged me without saying much.

"I love you, buddy," she said. "You be good."

"I love you too, Ma," I said. I hugged her once more.

My mother had made the trip with Rebekah's father, since she didn't like to travel alone and Gary wasn't about to take her. After she said goodbye to me, she climbed into the back seat of the van. As they drove away, she watched me through the back window for the entire length of the driveway. I saw her wipe a tear from her cheek.

I was more than ready to leave this last phase of my life behind.

As hard as it was for my mother to let go, I think she also knew that it was the only way for me to continue to change and grow. I'd already changed so much over the last year, since starting to find some sense of path and purpose. I was eager to explore where this burgeoning passion would take me. It was an uncertain new frontier, and for the first time I found myself running toward it rather than away.

My mother knew that, and I knew that she was proud.

216

CHAPTER 17

*O*NCE I HAD FINALLY ESCAPED, FOR REAL THIS TIME and not only in my head, it felt as if my life kicked into high gear. As painfully slow as my adolescence had at times seemed, my transition into early adulthood happened quickly. I had finally become unstuck and was now making up for lost time. In university, I opened up and found a whole new life. I followed my passions, I started to come out of my shell, and by my final year I had been elected student council president as well as the youngest-ever president of a provincial community mental health organization.

It wasn't always easy. I still experienced relapses in my depression, and thoughts of suicide occasionally crept back in. I couldn't just forget that old way of coping. However, I never acted on these thoughts again, and to a lesser or greater degree I coped. I continued to take medication, and I sought out help from the campus counselling services from time to time. However, being busy, being connected to others and having the clear goal of a degree to work toward helped. I had decided to study psychology, probably to better understand myself.

I was also finding my voice. During my third year, the university faculty went on strike just after Christmas. Being involved with the students' union by then, I believed that my job was to represent the interests of students, and I took it very seriously. The faculty union seemd to expect simple solidarity from the students, but to me it didn't make sense to advocate for higher salaries that were in part paid out of my growing student debt. I was also not particularly fond of being compliant anymore, and I overcompensated by becoming a contrarian instead.

There was a contentious five-week strike, and I came out of it with a sense that I wasn't especially popular among the professors in a wide variety of departments—including, most significantly for me, the psychology department. I was on track to complete all of the course requirements for an honours degree in psychology. When I eventually looked for professors in the psychology department to supervise my thesis, however, few would even answer my emails, and none agreed. When it seemed that my dream of completing a degree in psychology was at risk, I met with the department chair, a professor whom I admired. I explained my concerns.

"I get it," he said dismissively. "You want to do psychology because you had some issues and you want to understand them. Maybe you should try social work."

I had nothing against social work—social workers had been some of the most influential people in my recovery—but I was offended and discouraged. It is said that you should never meet your heroes, and I guess that's why. Heroes are never who you expect them to be, who you need them to be. This professor whom I had so admired, for both his intellect and his popularity, wasn't nearly as open-minded as I had hoped. However, with a whole new set of skills, I didn't stay down for long. The setback wasn't a trigger, as setbacks had been for me so many times before. Now it was motivating. I decided to find my own way and push through. If the existing structure doesn't work, build a new one.

I finished all of the course requirements for an honours degree in psychology anyway, except that without the thesis I wouldn't be recognized with the credentials to prove it. I ended up doing the same in philosophy, a field that was new to me but appealed to my theoretical side. I forged my own path between the two fields, bringing my five years of mostly psychology and philosophy courses together into an interdisciplinary honours project. I eventually cobbled together a small group of professors to supervise my thesis who, I think, took pity on me. I spent months immersed in Dante and Carl Jung, my twin academic passions, and these studies ended up shaping my entire view of mental illness and recovery. Both spoke to the idea of the journey to selfhood—a journey I'd been very actively exploring since my push through the treeline at the end of Gary's long driveway.

Dante's *Inferno* opens with him wandering, unsure of how he even got to where he is. Then he enters the gate to Hell.

"Abandon all hope, ye who enter here," reads the inscription above the entrance.

As Dante enters the gate and descends deeper, he discovers that Hell is a downward spiral. At the top, the damned are blown around helplessly in the wind. At the deepest, narrowest point of Hell, they're not burning in fire, they're encased in ice, immobilized for eternity, powerless. There are only a few in that lonely, cold, small, isolated place. That was exactly how my depression had felt.

But then Dante climbs past the ice. He escapes his Hell by following a small, winding stream, through a narrow, dark passageway, back up to the surface.

"From there we came out," Dante writes as he emerges from Hell, "to see, once more, the stars."

In many ways, Rebekah had been the one who helped me to emerge from Hell, to finally see the stars and not only the spaces between them. She was my high school sweetheart, and she had also already journeyed with me through all the very normal good and bad times of college.

So, I asked Rebekah to marry me. She said yes.

AFTER GRADUATION, I wasn't done figuring myself out. Big life changes still scared me—I needed routine—but stagnation scared me even more. I felt I had just started to find myself, and I wasn't ready to settle down just yet. Rebekah and I had talked about it, and we agreed that a long engagement probably made sense. We wanted to make sure we both had our degrees finished so we could start a life together properly.

In the five years that it took me to finish an undergraduate degree, Rebekah had completed both it and an education degree. I wanted the same opportunity to do more, but I'd been growing restless for the chance to do it on my own. I decided to pursue a Master of Science program in child development at the Erikson Institute in Chicago. I would move there without Rebekah. I still wanted to better understand my own childhood, and doing it through a graduate degree seemed a better long-term investment than many years of therapy. I was still very much focused on myself, and I had learned to substitute education as my escape.

It was never part of the plan for her to join me. This was something I felt I had to do by myself. She said she understood, but I knew she didn't. I knew that she felt abandoned. We ended up spending two years apart, though still together as a couple and talking nearly every day. It was a chance for me to try on yet another new life. Meanwhile, Rebekah moved in with her aunt and uncle in Prince Edward Island and began her new life as a teacher, separate from me.

One of the first major lessons I took away from my studies in Chicago was that children are hard-wired for struggle. That is, struggle is normal, because it helps people to learn who they are and how to be resilient. This was important for me to learn, because it helped me to realize that my childhood might not have been some major sob story after all, and that I wasn't screwed for life because of how I started. Maybe my upbringing was, actually, an advantage. This was a revelation to me. The past had passed. It was time to move on, let go and grow.

While I was living in Chicago, I started going to Argentine tango lessons. It was an impulse, an online coupon, that turned into a passion. Not only had I never taken a dance class before, dancing was one of the things I was most afraid of. I ended up returning almost every evening after that first class. The fact that I may have been motivated by terrible loneliness never really entered my mind, since that motivated a lot of things I did. My depression relapsed at least twice in grad school, but I more or less managed and kept it contained. I think that tango helped. Like Dante, it gave expression to my feelings when I still couldn't fully articulate them myself. In order to lead, I had to learn how to listen, and then learn the practical steps to communicate.

One night, I was walking back to my apartment after one of those lessons when I saw some rather inspirational graffiti scrawled across the sidewalk in thin lines of white paint.

Forgive yourself, it said.

I walked past those words, internalizing the message, every day.

...

WHILE I WAS living in Chicago, my mother moved out of Gary's house after another big fight. Nothing changes if nothing changes. She'd left him a few more times while I was in New Brunswick for undergrad. Since we had moved out together plenty of times before, I didn't expect this time to be any different. She always went back to him. The fight–flee–return was one of the predictable patterns of my childhood.

This time, however, she got herself an apartment. She'd never done that before. Her new apartment was on the other side of Nana Ag's duplex, the same one that her father had rented out to pay for the side of the house in which she was raised. It had become vacant, and sometimes all it takes to change everything is the right opportunity. She left this time, she said, to take care of her ailing mother, who had advanced dementia and was declining noticeably by the day. But a lot of people knew her real reasons.

With her own mother dying, Mom shared with me her growing concern about where she would end up once Gary eventually died. He was ten years older than her. She knew, she said, that he would leave everything to his kids. He had always made that clear. In their most recent fight, he had refused to show her his will. She wasn't even sure he had one, or if he had included her in it. Mom was convinced that Gary's kids would never allow her to keep living in their house once he was gone, despite the fact that she had lived there far longer than they did. So she finally left, as I did, and never moved back.

The next phase of her life was on my mother's mind a lot, because her retirement was only a few years away. Her life was changing, and I think she realized she could change with it or stay stuck. Although she had worked for almost thirty years in the same nursing settings, Mom switched into psychiatric nursing around the time she moved out of Gary's place. She worked on the ward where I had been held so many times a decade or so earlier.

Once Mom had a place she could really call her own, Rebekah and I visited and stayed with her the following Christmas. It was the first time in years I felt truly at home with my mother. She was happier than I had seen her in a long time. She had a new-found confidence, independence and freedom. She had finally escaped the isolation at the end of the dead-end dirt road.

She and Gary continued to see each other and were still in a relationship, but it was hard to describe exactly what their relationship was. It was awkward to call them boyfriend and girlfriend, since they'd been together, off and on, for over twenty years, and both seemed a little old for those labels anyway. He was just part of the fabric of her life, for better and worse.

Mom came to Chicago for my graduation in the summer of 2012. It was only the second flight she had ever taken. She was afraid to fly, but she did it anyway. All it takes to overcome fear is the right motivation on the other side.

When I was much younger, I remember her taking me to the end-of-term celebration when she completed a public speaking course. Mom was terribly afraid of public speaking, but she wanted to take this course to try to overcome her fear. In the short, prepared speech she gave to the assembled group of a few dozen friends and family—each of the participants had to give a speech, but hers was the only one I remembered—she talked about her fear of flying, and how painfully her ears had popped on her one trip. She beamed, her face red, as she came back to her seat from the front of the room, obviously proud that she had overcome at least one fear that night. I didn't think much of it as a kid. It took me more than twenty years to be proud of her for that.

She told me how proud she was of me, too, as I prepared to walk across the stage to accept my graduate degree. The two-year adventure seemed to be over in a blink. I had packed more living and new experiences into that time than I ever had before. I was starting to feel a certain gratitude for my struggle. I didn't like many things that had happened to me, but I now knew that the events of my life only have the meaning I give them. Learning is what you do with the things done to you.

But what I saw in myself as endless curiosity and ambition, Rebekah saw as a restless heart. She was the exact opposite of me at this point in her life. She craved stability, and the uncertainty that now gave me energy triggered a lot of anxiety in her. She saw "starting over" as never getting ahead, while I saw it as wiping the slate clean. So, as we were planning our wedding from two different countries, we decided we would build a new life together in Toronto as a compromise.

Throughout our long-distance wedding planning, my mother was a consistent and grounding support for us. She repeatedly reminded us, and the many others who felt compelled to share their advice, that it was our wedding and we should do what made us happy. She hid her own anxieties, especially relating to her poor self-image. She couldn't make up her mind about her dress, so she bought two. She ended up wearing the one she didn't like, because the one that she loved matched the wedding party and she didn't want to draw any attention to herself. Blessed are the peacemakers, and all that.

We were married in July 2012. I had no idea I could ever be that happy.

We settled in Toronto. As fall came, the happiness started to wilt, as happiness does if left untended. Not our happiness together, but mine with myself. I had developed a persistent fear that the next relapse would be worse than the last. Maybe the next one would be the big one. Although I had never since been as ill as I was that night I went to the bridge, before being saved by the stranger in the light-brown jacket, I still feared that would be my ultimate fate. If happiness is temporary and recovery is contingent and in cyclical flux, then maybe it too is destined to end. Nothing lasts forever.

"It won't always be like this," I said aloud to myself.

I sat in the car before starting another shift at the minimum-wage retail job I had to get in order to pay the rent. I hadn't gotten a job I had interviewed for before we moved, so I had sent out dozens of resumés to try to find work in the mental health field, but with little or no response.

When I finally did get a job, it was on my third attempt, at the local branch of the Canadian Mental Health Association. I had interviewed for two different positions, but they hired me for a third one. I became a case manager, helping sixteen-to-twenty-four-year-olds navigate the disjointed, inadequate, Byzantine mental health system. I didn't really have much formal clinical training to speak of, but I learned quickly that wasn't what these young people were looking for anyway. They wanted someone who could listen, believe them, support them and, if needed, help them find the more intensive clinical interventions they required. It helped that I had been in a similar position to many of them not all that long ago, though I knew my role, and appreciated the difference between my situation and theirs.

As Christmas approached, that financial security allowed Rebekah and me to start building our own traditions and foundations of family. We had decided to spend the holidays at our new home in Toronto rather than going back to Cape Breton that year. Rebekah was still working at a toy store, hoping someday to get a job as a teacher, while I now held down both my case worker job and the retail sales associate job on evenings and weekends. It was hard, but we were making it work.

One evening, I came home from another late shift and Rebekah was sitting on our little second-hand couch. I could sense her nervousness as soon as I opened the door. When I came in and rounded the corner to see her, she was holding a little wrapped gift she had bought me. As I sat down and opened the gift, it became clear. Inside the box were two of the tiniest onesies I had ever seen, each embroidered with the word "Daddy."

My heart pounded and I felt a flush of warmth. "Are we ready?" I managed to choke out, through tears.

"I don't know," she responded. "Are you happy?"

"I am," I said with a quivering smile. I ran my fingers over the stitching on the tiny hat.

"Is it okay that I'm scared?" I asked. I felt like a little kid about to enter a dark room.

"I'm scared too," she told me. "But we'll be okay."

I didn't want to tell her how afraid I really was.

I didn't want to tell her why I was so afraid.

"My children might be just like me," I had once said to Heather, the social worker in the basement psychiatric ward that held me under twenty-four-hour observation.

That, I still thought, would be a catastrophe.

NOAH WAS due on September 11.

He stayed where he was longer than planned. Even by September 20, 2013, he was showing no desire to separate from his mother. An induction and delivery date was scheduled, and we were to wait for the call to report to the hospital.

My mother had come to stay with us to share in the moment and offer her support. Nana Ag had finally died a little over a month earlier. She had a long, slow decline through dementia, with my mother by her side the whole way. Mom was devastated to lose her mother; the whole family was. They asked me to come home to Cape Breton to speak at the funeral. I said a few words before the start of the mass and ended with a poem by John Henry Newman:

When in due lines her Saviour dear
His scatter'd saints shall range,
And knit in love souls parted here,
Where cloud is none, nor change.

The call for the induction came when I was at work. It was around 3 p.m. We met at the hospital less than an hour later. I marvelled at how easy it was to tell which parts of the hospital got the most donations. The maternity wing curved and swooped in comforting, soft angles of glass and wood. Cancer research and treatment had its own state-of-the-art building, scientific and advanced-looking. The psychiatric treatment areas were spread through an old brick building that looked as though it had endured a war, with dirty carpet throughout, tiny offices with only partially working air conditioners retrofitted into the windows facing the parking lot, and the unmistakable stench of depression.

We settled into the birthing room and met a parade of professionals, all very soft-spoken. Late into the night, there still wasn't much progress. My mother had been sitting in one of the big chairs near the window, occasionally scribbling down notes on a little pad of paper.

"What's that?" I asked.

"It's so you have something to remember all this when it's over," she said.

I looked over her shoulder and saw her familiar nursing shorthand.

17:51—Oxytocin Drip started @ 2
18:14—Drip ↑ 4
18:45—Drip ↑ 6
19:05—Drip ↑ 8
20:37—Drip ↑ 12
20:55—+++ uncomfortable
22:25—Drip ↑ 14 as if contractions weren't hard enough

At quarter to four in the morning, twelve hours after we arrived at the front door, the doctor and his team were called back into the operating room for the delivery. Rebekah was told to push, but not much seemed to be happening. By the fifth set of pushes, she was exhausted.

"I can't," she cried. "I can't do it."

"Yes, you can, Beckie," my mother said. She had been introduced to her as Beckie and even a decade later never called her anything else. "You can do it."

At 4:12 a.m., Rebekah managed one more push, and with it I watched the rest of Noah's body emerge. A rush of release washed through my body as well, as if I could feel some small part of what she was experiencing. Noah's skin was dusty grey. The umbilical cord was wrapped twice around his neck. The doctor showed his student, then with two fingers slipped it up over his face and off his head with one fluid motion. They clamped and cut the cord, then took him away quickly.

"Why isn't he crying?" Rebekah asked in a tired, worried voice.

"They just have to clean his mouth and nose," I lied, with authority. In my head, I had never prayed so hard to hear someone cry.

After two long minutes, he did. From a small table across the room, where he was surrounded by two or three blue-gowned people, Noah cried. I was overcome by the sound of this fragile new life crying with every ounce of unfamiliar air in his little lungs. He had finally discovered a whole new world. This world apart from his mother was scary and strange. They brought him over and placed him on Rebekah's chest. I came in close and cradled his tiny head in my hand. Mom stood back and watched me, in an instant, change from a son into a father.

I looked up at her, and she was crying too.

FIVE DAYS after the birth of my son, I delivered a TEDx Talk on suicide.

I wanted to do it because I wanted to expose people to a different way of thinking about suicide. I wanted to do it not as an expert, because I wasn't, but from the perspective of my lived experience of recovery. The truth was, I still struggled from time to time. Still, I wanted to challenge people and help them to understand what goes through someone's mind during a life-and-death crisis.

On the day of my talk, after months of preparation, just before I stepped out onto the big red dot in the middle of the stage, I had a panic attack. My speaking coach found me, brought me to a small area, a tiny, dark space, between two doors backstage.

"I want you to go through your talk with me," he said. "Not the script, just the ideas."

I didn't want to let go of the script. That was my security blanket. But I trusted him. Over the next ten minutes, in that small, dark hallway, we un-memorized my talk, and I learned, a little more, to let go.

When I emerged and stepped onstage, the first people I saw in the audience were Rebekah and my mother. Our five-day-old baby was with Rebekah's grandmother and my mother's sisters at a hotel a block away. I planted my feet—they didn't move for the next fifteen minutes—and I spoke my truth.

In many ways, it was a truth I was still experiencing at that moment. The audience responded with a loud, emotional standing ovation. Before I left the stage, I looked at my wife in the audience, and my mother sitting next to her. They were smiling, and theirs was the only applause I heard.

THE TALK quickly became a viral hit. Over the next year, I received messages from people all over the world. Their stories became familiar to me: they were sorry for contacting me but they needed someone to talk to, and after seeing the talk, they felt they could talk to me. Most of them said they felt that nobody else had understood them until they saw my talk. It was all very flattering, and overwhelming. It also made me feel like an imposter.

"Who am I to tell people how to get better?" I thought. "I haven't even figured it out for myself yet." I was also a new parent, but in a lot of ways I still felt as though I needed parenting myself.

We had no family in Toronto who could help us, and we hadn't made many close friends yet. So we spent a lot of time trying to reconnect with our own families. We took Noah home to

Cape Breton for his first Christmas—we still called Cape Breton "home"—and that helped us to refill on our need for family. We stayed at my mother's apartment. Although Mom had used the need to care for Nana Ag as the excuse to move out of Gary's house, she continued living on her own after her mother died. That's how we knew it was for good this time. She and Gary were still seeing each other, but she seemed happier than ever to no longer be living in a common-law relationship.

We were eager to establish our own family traditions, so Rebekah and I knew this would probably be our last Christmas there. We took time to see everyone. Krista and her husband had three kids. Raymond was in a stable relationship in Halifax but came down for the holidays. Dad was still scrapping cars, living at his mother's, and Nana Marg was as fierce as ever. She quit smoking for a while, after having a heart attack and ending up on the edge of death. Dad found her on the floor and administered CPR as best he could from what he had seen on daytime television. She lived, and was back up to two packs a day.

It was the best Christmas we'd ever had. It was filled with lots of laughter and love, and a few tears. Mom had always cried whenever the choir at Holy Redeemer sang "Amazing Grace" because it reminded her of her dad. Now she also cried when they sang "Gentle Woman," a hymn about the Holy Mother, because the grief over the loss of her own mother was still so present. That Christmas, at least, I was there to hold her hand as she cried. Not all problems can be fixed. Sometimes all you can do is hold hands.

By the time Noah's first birthday came in September, it seemed like only yesterday that we were gowned in the operating room, anxious and exhausted, praying for him to cry. Now we had spent many sleepless nights hoping he wouldn't. We flew my mother in to celebrate and to stay with us for a few days. She was starting to enjoy travelling, now that she had the opportunity to do it more. She would be turning fifty-five in November, and was eligible for early retirement, so she talked about travel as something she would like to do to occupy her time.

Mom had come a long way in the years since her public speaking class in the church basement, where she spoke about her fear of flying. We'd all come a long way from who we once were. Still, she seemed quieter than usual on that trip. It was just after the one-year anniversary of her own mother's death, and I knew that she missed her.

It was a sunny late September morning when my mother and I took Noah for a walk. He was asleep in his stroller as we entered Mount Pleasant Cemetery through the east gate. Mom commented that a graveyard was a strange place to go for a walk. She soon changed her mind when she saw the pristine landscaping, winding pathways and impressive architecture of its many monuments.

We ambled along, not really in a hurry to go anywhere, passing a row of ostentatious tombs that bore the names of some of Canada's wealthiest families. Mom lingered a bit at a few. We talked about death. I knew it had been on her mind a lot over the last year. My mother talked about how she didn't want to be forgotten. I promised her that would never happen. I reminded her, as I did when we had danced to Nat King Cole at our wedding reception, that she was "Unforgettable." She went home a few days later.

After she did, I felt an unexpected urge. I suddenly wanted to find the stranger in the light-brown jacket—the man who saved my life all those years ago on the overpass between Sydney and Whitney Pier. The desire to find him had been there for a while. It started as dreams, when I was living in Chicago, scribbled down early in the morning in a journal I kept beside my bed. But then something made the desire bubble over and turn into an imperative. I had been talking about him for years in telling my story, but in truth, I didn't actually know if he was real. Our encounter was so short, and I was in such a closed-down place in my mind, that I worried I had made him up as some kind of protective mechanism or false memory. I hadn't yet learned which thoughts to trust and which to question.

Unable to trust my subjective experience, I brought my analytical mind to the problem. I needed independent verification that the man existed. I reached out to a few journalists for some tips on how to do this kind of investigative research. I requested the police records from the relevant local department, and then submitted a formal Freedom of Information Act request when they refused.

I visited Cape Breton in November 2014 to see what else I could find. I planned to appeal the police decision not to disclose my records. Mom drove with me to the station and waited in the car while I went in to drop off the paperwork. She didn't say much about it to me. I almost felt that she was apprehensive that if I went digging around too much in my past, I might not like what I found. Maybe she worried I might get stuck there again. Spending too much time cracking open the history books of your life can have that kind of impact.

By the new year, there was still no response from the police department. Mom was disappointed that we hadn't come back home for Christmas but seemed to understand our need to start making an independent life for ourselves. Although she was enjoying her own independence, she also never fully got over her empty nest syndrome. Between my sister's three kids and my one, she filled the void with her grandkids. She talked to Noah on the phone a few times a week and, since my sister and her family still lived just up the street, Mom often had the grandkids over to stay the night.

On January 24, my sister's then eight-year-old daughter Brooklyn stayed over with my mom. The next day, she came downstairs to have some lunch that my mother was preparing for her. When she reached the bottom of the stairs, she found Mom on the floor between the kitchen and the living room. She was convulsing violently, her face twisted, her lips and fingertips turning blue. Brooklyn called her mother, who panicked.

"There's something wrong with Nanny," Brooklyn said, crying.

Krista rushed to the house, where she found Mom still unconscious on the floor, struggling to breathe. The convulsions had stopped by then, but her face was still contorted in a way that was seared into my sister's memory. She repositioned Mom on her side, which seemed to help her breathe better, and called an ambulance.

When the ambulance finally arrived, Mom was still unconscious. She was taken to hospital and placed in isolation. My sister called me after Mom had been stabilized.

"Don't worry, but Mom had another seizure this morning," she said.

"Okay, how is she doing now?" I asked.

"She's doing better. She's still kind of out of it and can't really talk yet," Krista answered.

"Should I come home?" I asked.

"Just wait, I think she's okay now," she answered.

None of this was new to us. Mom had been having a seizure every few years for as long as I could remember, so it didn't cause us as much worry as it might have if it had never happened before. The first one happened shortly after my father left. They came a few times when she was living with Gary, always while she was asleep in bed. The theory at the time was that the seizures were caused either by stress or by her sleep apnea, which was restricting her oxygen while she slept. At least, that had been the theory up until the most recent seizure before this one, which happened while she was fully awake at work. She was filling medications for her nursing rounds when a seizure overtook her, causing her to fall hard on the concrete floor. She was surrounded by doctors within seconds that time, and recovered quickly.

This time was different. This time seemed more serious. Something had changed. She wasn't breathing for longer periods of time, her face seemed twisted for longer, and she was unconscious for longer. A series of tests was performed, many of which I was familiar with from having had my own seizures. A spot on the inside of her skull, on her forehead just above her left eye, had been discovered years ago. She had been having annual MRI scans to monitor it ever since. The spot was a calcification resulting from the way a decades-old head injury had healed, like scar tissue made of bone on the inside surface of her forehead. It never seemed to change, but they were keeping an eye on it just in case. I hated how inept and lazy the health care system in my hometown seemed but also recognized that my own bad experience was probably colouring my perception.

Mom was released from hospital after a few days where they still hadn't found or fixed anything. That's when I started asking, then practically begging, for her to come to Toronto.

"We can get you in to see a specialist at one of the big hospitals here, an epilepsy clinic," I told her. "We can finally figure out what's going on. If we figure it out, we can fix it."

"I don't want anyone poking around inside my head," she demurred.

...

Mom was out of hospital by the time Bell Let's Talk day came around at the end of January. I'm always very active on this annual social media campaign to raise awareness for mental health, and was especially so that year. I hadn't been seeing any progress through bureaucratic channels in my search for the stranger in the light-brown jacket who saved my life, so I started a conversation with a producer at *Canada AM*, Canada's long-standing morning show at the time. I had appeared on the show a couple of times already to talk about other mental health issues, and I had worked with a number of the producers and hosts at the network.

I had been seeing over the years how much more effective it was to get things done through social action and public discourse, as opposed to waiting for change. I told the producer that I wanted to come on and ask for the public's help in finding the man who saved me, and that I wanted to do it the day after Bell Let's Talk. They sent a car for me very early the next morning, and it was still dark when I arrived at the studio. We did the live interview, in which I told some of my story, and they showed clips of my TED Talk. After leaving, in the car that was taking me back home, I sent out a tweet and a Facebook post asking for the public's help.

The story didn't take long to go viral around the world.

As a result, it only took about eight hours to produce results. By that afternoon I had been contacted by two men who said they knew who I was talking about. The first one said that he was my stranger's roommate at the time, and that he had come home after it happened and told him about it. The other one said he was the brother of the stranger's girlfriend, basically his brother-in-law, and that they shared the story among the family and knew him as a hero. The former said he had seen my TED Talk about a week earlier. When he saw it, he sent it to the stranger to watch, believing I was talking about him.

Coincidentally, a week before anyone, except a handful of people, knew that I was looking for him, the stranger in the light-brown jacket had started writing me a letter in case someday he found me. Now, the brother-in-law asked if the stranger could send me the letter he had written. I agreed, suddenly afraid, feeling the familiar sensation of not knowing what I had gotten myself into.

The letter arrived by email a short time later. It sat in my email inbox for hours, unread, as I tried to slow time down and adjust to the change. Adjusting to change takes a little longer after you've had an adjustment disorder, even long into recovery. The best way I had learned to adjust was just to do it, and do it, and do it again.

Around midnight, I summoned up the courage to read the letter. I flicked on the camera on my iPad. I figured that I had started this story in public, so I might as well finish it there too. I opened the email.

Hi there,

My name is Mike Richey. I live in Halifax, and work at a crisis center for at-risk youth from across the province. I started my career as a Youth Care Worker about 13 years ago in my hometown of Sydney. At the time, I was working at the Boys Residential Center in New Waterford. I was on my way to a backshift (12am–8am) one night, driving over the overpass. I remember there were no other cars on the road or anyone else around. As I drove, I could see what appeared to be a person standing on the opposite side of the railing looking down. My immediate thought was "that's not good."

I drove to the end of the overpass and ran into the first open convenience store. I told the clerk that someone might be trying to jump off the overpass and to please call the police. He was doing so as I ran out of the store, got back into my car, and drove back to the person. Although you're not supposed to stop on the overpass, I parked my car and began to walk towards the person. As I approached, I could see it was a teenage boy. I didn't want to startle him or overwhelm him, so I gave him lots of space. I acknowledged that things didn't seem to be going so well, and kept the conversation light. I wanted him to know I wasn't there to judge or change his mind about things, I was just there to listen.

He didn't talk much, and I didn't push the conversation. There were a lot of long pauses where the only sound was the ice-cold wind blowing in my ears. I asked him his name and he told me it was Mark. We continued to talk as a single police car approached and parked a distance away. A female officer walked towards us and also established communication while maintaining distance as well. We talked to Mark for what felt like hours (although it wasn't). To this day I have no idea how long we were up there. It was as if time stood still.

At some point along the way, more police cars arrived, as well as paramedics on both sides of the overpass. Onlookers began to gather. Everyone was kept a safe distance away. As we talked, we asked Mark if we could move a little bit closer to him so we could hear him better. Mark took a moment, then nodded in agreement. As I stood next to him, I looked directly over the railing, seeing things from his perspective for the first time. I felt sick. As I stood safely on one side, Mark was on the other with just the heels of his shoes holding him up on the ledge. He was keeping his balance on the railing by the tips of his fingers. I remember thinking "if anything goes wrong . . . a gust of wind . . . a loss of footing . . . I'm going to watch this boy fall to his death." Mark began to repeat how he "tried" and "can't do it anymore." He wouldn't elaborate, just kept repeating "I tried . . . I tried . . ." I felt like he was working himself up to let go.

I was completely focused on his fingers, waiting for them to start slipping. Within moments, they did, and as he leaned forward into nothing, I reached out and put my arm around his chest. The officer quickly grabbed him by the back of his jacket. We both pulled him backwards over the railing. Mark was safe. Paramedics rushed in and he was taken away to the hospital. I gave the police a brief statement and was on my way, never to see Mark again.

The events of that night have stuck with me for 12 years. It was difficult for me to process, and it took a long time before I could get past it. I've shared the story with those close to me over the years, always saying I wish I knew where that boy was today. I wondered if he ever went back and finished what he was attempting to do that night. I wondered if he ever found the peace he was looking for. All I could do was remain optimistic and hope for the latter.

Fast forward 12 years. I'm at work and a friend of mine sends me a text. We were roommates at the time of the events on the overpass, and he knew the story. He said "I just watched this TED talk . . . I think he's talking about you . . ." I went to the washroom to have some privacy as I watched the video. As I stood there holding my phone, I was overwhelmed with emotion. I listened to this man talk about being on the overpass that night as a youth, and I was suddenly back there again. Mark had grown up. I was looking at this successful, professional, confident man, who was using his experiences in life to help others. I began to cry. I never knew you could feel so proud of someone you spent such a brief moment in time with. I got myself together *and finished my shift, although my head was elsewhere for the rest of the night.*

That was about a week ago. Since then I've been contemplating contacting you. My biggest concern was that you would like to keep things the way they are. I didn't know if you wanted to keep "the man in the light brown jacket" anonymous and didn't feel like it was my place to make that decision for you. Then I saw your interview yesterday on Canada AM, and your tweets about wanting to find the man from that night. I knew it was time to write this letter.

Mike

CHAPTER 18

FINALLY, THIS PERSON, THIS NAMELESS STRANGER WHO I wasn't even sure was real, who had been such an important part of my story for so long, had a name. If he had a name, that meant he was real after all. If he was real, then it meant that my story, my memories, my feelings were too. That might seem like a given to anyone who trusts how they feel and has certainty around the story they tell themselves about their life. For me, however, this was life-changing.

At once, I was glad to have filled in a missing piece of myself. I was also apprehensive. Mike had become a major talking point for me. I think I had turned him into a character, a player in the drama in my head. What if the real Mike was nothing like the stranger I had written about and talked about onstage? What if he didn't match up to the impressive monument of him I had built in my mind?

Worse—what if he didn't like me?

After we reconnected by email and the attention died down, Mike and I started to talk about how we could meet in person. I knew that I couldn't properly express my gratitude over email;

it had to be face to face. Still, I had no idea how I actually would thank him. How do you thank someone not only for saving your life but for giving you your entire life? Ever since he saved me, I had been modelling my own journey on my choice to be like him: the stranger who noticed people, who had their back, who reached out rather than shouted from the sidelines.

The journey to find him also made me think a lot about my past. I had sensed uncertainty from my mother when we were in the police station parking lot, as I was requesting my police records and starting the search for the stranger in the light-brown jacket. Maybe that uncertainty wasn't entirely unfounded, and maybe I really wasn't ready to go digging around in my head. I had been running from it all this time, after all. And I realized that, up to and including the brief time it took to search for and reconnect with Mike, I had started to relapse yet again. Sometimes I still didn't see it coming, and it took an outside event like this to make me realize what was happening. Recovery is strange and non-linear like that.

After I found Mike, things started to slowly turn around. Filling in this hole in my narrative made me feel more coherent, less of a fraud. I didn't know how to thank him for giving me my whole life, so I thought that the best I could do was to show him some of the life that he had given me. I flew him up to Toronto in the spring. Since I had kicked off my search for him in such a public way, and we reconnected with public attention too, we were joined in our reunion by a *Canada AM* crew. We met, on camera, in downtown Toronto. When we saw each other in person, for the first time since that other first time, he wrapped his arms around me. That was also like the other first time. I introduced him to Rebekah, and to my little boy. I showed him some of the life I had built, which, while by no means perfect, I would never have believed possible for myself when I was standing on the edge of that overpass.

That idea first came to me while I was on a short trip home to Cape Breton for a speaking engagement in March 2015. That was before Mike and I had planned to meet in person but after we started talking by email. I arrived late at night. The university that was sponsoring my talk put me up in a hotel, as event sponsors usually did. I called my mother as soon as I landed. I knew she expected I would come and stay at her apartment.

"Mom," I said, "I'm going to stay at the hotel tonight. I don't want you to have to wait up too late." I explained that there was no sense in wasting the hotel room, but I'm not sure that was the real reason. I think part of me just wanted my own space. It was still hard for me to be in the same small city where so much of my trauma lived. I could process it when I was far away, but when it was next door, it was more difficult.

"Okay, that's fine," she said, sounding disappointed.

The next morning, I checked out of the hotel and went to my mother's place to spend the rest of the short stay with her. I didn't want to stay long.

This was going to be the first time I had spoken to a hometown audience since I left all those years ago and went on to find some relative success. Expectations were high, and a good chunk of the audience was probably going to be related to me in some way. Mom would be there, and Dad and Gary. Mike's mother, Sherry, was also going to attend. I was feeling overwhelmed but had developed a certain comfort with that feeling over the years. Stress seemed to encourage my creative impulsivity now, rather than the destructive impulsivity it triggered before. I had learned to tap into my stress, to redirect it toward something more helpful.

A local journalist got in touch, wanting to do another story on my search for Mike and on my talk that evening. We filmed an interview, talking about how important this journey had been to me. By that point I'd done so many of these interviews that it was starting to feel scripted.

"It might be your hundredth time saying it," I was once told, "but it's probably someone else's first time hearing it." That helped to put things in perspective.

I emailed the journalist back after the interview and told her I had an idea. I was kind of winging it, as usual. I asked if she would be interested in coming back to the overpass with me, back to the exact spot where I climbed the railing and attempted to jump. She responded in less than a minute.

"Yes, absolutely," she said.

I was sitting in my mother's living room, with her and her sister Mary. We were laughing and telling stories of their adventures when they had visited me over the years in New Brunswick, Chicago and Toronto. It triggered me to reflect on how I wasn't the same struggling kid I used to be. My life was no longer defined by my past. I was still in charge of my own story. Even though that was the same realization that had kick-started my recovery in earnest, as I waited for the taxi outside the hospital all those years ago, I still needed to be reminded from time to time.

"Mom," I said, "I'm going to be meeting up with a reporter in about an hour."

"Okay," she answered. She was sitting across from me, on the edge of the black faux leather couch, with her hands between her knees.

"Would you come with me?" I asked. It was an impulse. I hadn't planned on coming to Cape Breton to reconcile my mother's experience of my struggle, as a parent trying to understand her suicidal son. I was just trusting that I could ride the waves of my feelings rather than be swept away and drowned by them.

"Yeah, for what?" she answered.

"Well, I'm going to walk back over the overpass, and the reporter is going to come." She shifted in her seat. "You wouldn't have to say or do anything, just come along."

"I guess so." She hesitated. "My hair is a mess. And I look fat. And this jacket is old."

"Mom, you look fine. You'll hardly be in the shot anyway." I actually had no idea what the reporter would want to do, but I could tell she was anxious. I knew my mother well enough to know that she wanted to do it but was self-conscious. I knew because I had learned these behaviours from her. I felt the same inhibition inside nearly every day, every time I stepped onstage or in front of a camera. I had learned to identify it, make friends with it, push through it. The nervous feeling in my gut became my compass for where I needed to push myself harder.

"You don't have to if you don't want to," I told her, "but I would like you to come if you can."

"Okay, I will," she said.

About an hour later, we met the reporter at a convenience store parking lot. In retrospect, I realize it was the same place where Mike had stopped to get the clerk to call 911 a dozen years earlier. Once her camera was set up, she followed Mom and me as we walked the short distance to the overpass. I walked this same route the night I was going there to kill myself. It was a chilly March day, just like that other time, with wet snow still covering the ground and a sharp wind blowing. We came to the spot, just before the three tall old wooden electrical poles connected by a rusty steel X-shaped brace.

I looked down and saw the drop. I started to cry, unexpectedly.

The concrete edge, the ground below—it all looked different now. It didn't look as far down as I remembered. It was about forty feet, max, from rail to ground. According to experts, the statistical chance of dying from that height is under 50 percent. There's a wide margin: people have fallen ten feet, broken their necks and died, while one man fell eighteen thousand feet from a plane with a defective parachute and survived with only a sprained leg. Maybe a lot depends on the landing. Then again, I thought about how Gary fell at least twenty feet and landed directly on his head but survived. Of course, he changed, but who isn't changed by their trauma?

I didn't know much about statistics when I was fifteen. I was sure then that a headfirst fall would have the intended outcome. The view from the bridge was different now, too, compared with what it was when I was standing on the edge. Almost all of the old buildings were gone. Everything looked so much cleaner now. A lush green space spread out before me, newly landscaped but as yet unfinished, with a few fledgling saplings planted here and there. The problem with living entirely in your mind is that it's decorated by memories. Memories are static, but life moves and changes. Things collapse, others are torn down, still others grow anew. If I let them.

My hands were resting on the top railing. When I felt the cold steel under my fingers, I was back in that moment. It was not a memory or a story—I was there again. My mother was standing next to me this time, though.

Jump, you coward, the stranger on the sidelines said with a laugh. I can better distinguish between the voices in my head these days. That is big progress for me. Some are voices from memories, others dreams, others still demons. There are doctors, nurses, parents, priests in there too. The voice of my saviour-stranger, Mike, from over my shoulder. One voice is mine. I try to listen to that one the most now.

Mom put her left hand over my right, blocking the cold wind. I looked down and saw her familiar touch, her wrinkles. There were more of them than I remembered. Life moves. Mom had always been the same age in my memory. Suddenly we were both older. I turned to her, put my head on her shoulder. I let the tears stay in my eyes.

"You've come so far, Mark," she said.

I forgot about the camera, which was still watching us from about ten feet away. I think she did too. It was so windy, the microphone I was wearing didn't pick up anything we said.

"I'm not sure sometimes, Ma," I admitted. I felt guilty for everything I had put her through. That feeling of guilt started when I became a parent myself. I still felt I should have my shit together by now. I had no reason not to—look at all I had accomplished and overcome and had to look forward to. My life seemed so great now. So why did I still feel this way sometimes?

"I know, buddy," she said. "I know you're not." Nobody knew me like my mother. "But you have. Look at everything you've done, and you're just getting started," she went on. "You're going to change the world. I'm so proud of you."

"I love you, Mom," I answered. I was apologizing, finally, for everything.

"I love you too," she replied, and she knew.

Love speaks in forgiveness.

THAT NIGHT, I did the hometown talk. Turnout was good, and everyone who showed up seemed to know me already. I met Mike's mom and introduced her to my own mother. The talk was tight; I'd learned to evaluate the talks by my control of the narrative and the engagement of the room. It was an easy and friendly room to engage.

I spent the next day visiting with family. Mom and I went to breakfast with Gary, and we teased him about how long Mom had been in his life versus his original family.

"You know, Gary," I said, "technically, we've been in your life for more than twice as long as your ex-wife was." The point, though maybe not charitable, was clear. We still felt, always felt, second-class. We might as well find it funny. Comedy is tragedy plus time.

Mom teased him about it for the rest of our breakfast. We knew that it made him uncomfortable. Mom and I both felt that he'd never really moved on. Life moves on, but not everybody or everything moves on with it.

Static people and places don't have to keep us stuck with them. Instead, I'd learned, they can be a reference for how far we ourselves have moved. Growth is relative. Mom and I had grown so much, relatively. I think that's why we laughed, not at him, but at ourselves. We found happiness on the other side of struggle by going through it, not around it. We had climbed through Hell and emerged different on the other side.

I went to bed that night happy after a surprisingly fulfilling visit. The next time I opened my eyes, my 3 a.m. alarm was ringing. I had to get to the airport for my 5:30 a.m. flight. My mother emerged from her room as I rounded the corner by the little bathroom. I told her to go back to bed, but there was no point. She was used to getting up that early anyway. We went downstairs and gathered my things by the door.

Before I left, Mom ran upstairs to get something for me. She came back down a minute later. "I want you to have these," she said. "They belonged to my father." She handed me a set of black rosary beads.

I had been thinking about visiting the overpass for my own closure. I hadn't thought the moment would be as meaningful for my mother. She later told my sister how she finally felt at peace with everything that had happened. She had blamed herself for my struggles; maybe it was her fault, maybe she had been a bad mother. For years, she lived in fear of losing me. She went to work in the psych ward, after so many years of working everywhere else, to finally understand. What I understood as her forgiveness was also her apology. She didn't have to be afraid anymore, and neither did I. It was never her fault. She, like I, was doing her best with the hand she'd been dealt. Life wasn't what she had planned, but plans change, so you change with them.

Before I left, I hugged her. She was trying not to cry. We'd done this routine dozens of times over the years, and she cried every time. Some things never change.

I got in the driver's seat of the car and started to pull away. When I looked back, as I always did, Mom was still standing there at the door in her white pyjamas. I waved goodbye. She wiped her eye quickly, then waved back.

I drove away slowly before sunrise. I felt an unexpected lump in my throat, the burning of tears in my eyes. I judged myself harshly for it. *Be a man.* Habits are hard to kill. But then I self-corrected my self-judgment.

"It's not weird to love your mother," I said out loud.

My mind is a collection of voices. Some voices speak unbidden from memory. I remembered the sidewalk graffiti that I walked past every day in Chicago.

Forgive yourself, it said.

CHAPTER 19

You don't realize how far you've come until you're forced to look back.

The morning of July 1, 2015, started slowly. All the media attention over the reunion of Mike and me had moved on. I had celebrated my twenty-eighth birthday, my speaking engagements were regular and frequent, and I had continued to travel a lot. Following the realization of my relapse, and all of the changes to my life that had happened over the preceding spring, I was still not fully myself.

It was Canada Day, around 7 a.m., and we were getting ready to go on a picnic like the one our little family had enjoyed together the year before. We didn't really want to go but needed something to lift the fog of sadness that Rebekah and I were feeling. The morning before, we had had to take one of our two cats to the vet to be euthanized. His health had been declining for several weeks as his kidneys failed. On the morning of June 30, it was clear that we couldn't ask him to continue for our sake anymore.

I had bought Pepper as a five-week-old kitten when I was a high school student, on my second summer study trip to Quebec between grades eleven and twelve. He had moved around a lot with me over the years, from the times we had to flee from Gary's home to the time he lived with Rebekah and then moved with us when we went to college in Fredericton. He came with me when I moved to Chicago, and then when I moved back to Toronto to settle down.

Pepper was euthanized in a small, quiet room a few blocks from where we lived in Toronto. When the quick procedure was finished, the vet showed Rebekah and me some brochures for various urns and boxes, cremations and burials, and we indicated which would be most suitable. I found myself wrestling with two competing thoughts:

"This is silly, it was just a cat," on one side. "He's dead now, and none of this matters."

"He was my childhood friend, and I miss him," on the other.

I was sad for the end of our story together. This little animal had witnessed most of the tragedy and comedy of my life for more than a decade. He had played with me when I was happy and cuddled me when I was sad. I dreaded the loss of our connection more than the loss of a pet. He was one of the last remaining pieces of my past.

On the short walk back to our apartment building, as we approached the front entrance, I stopped and turned to Rebekah.

"You know," I said, "I can't remember the last time that I really grieved."

The death of my grandmother had made me sad, but she had been declining for many years. Most of that time I visited only once or twice a year. By the time she died, well into dementia, she wasn't the same grandmother I had grown up with. She'd forgotten us all for good, even my mother, who along with Aunt Mary bathed and fed her, gave her her medications and listened for her stirrings late into the night. As hard as it was for my mother to be Nana Ag's caretaker, she missed her mom desperately.

I think that grief is our resistance to letting go of the future rather than the past. Grief is what hard change feels like. If we do it well, we come out different, better, regardless of the change. If we resist, we're changed anyway, but more painfully. In the case of my grandmother, many of us had the chance to grieve her before she died. The future is less scary if we think we know what's going to happen, based on our interpretation of what already has. When we lose that certainty, we lose our safety.

"It's not supposed to be this way" holds us back. It's a rigid way of thinking that collapses all possibility. It's a judgment based more on what we want than on what is. It's how I felt on the bridge.

Later that evening, as we sat on the couch watching Noah play with his toys, my mother called. She had seen a picture of Pepper that I had posted to Facebook, with a caption expressing my sadness at his loss. She called to comfort me.

"I thought he was doing better," she said.

"He was for a while," I replied. "When we woke up this morning, we knew that it was his time."

"I'm sorry, buddy," she said in her comforting voice, if a little tired-sounding.

As we did a few times a week, I put the call on speakerphone and handed the phone over to Noah. Imitating someone—we never really determined who—he held the cellphone on his shoulder with his head cocked to one side, leaving his hands free to gesture. They talked for a few minutes about simple things—how he was doing and what his plans were for tomorrow. He couldn't really answer yet, it was mostly just babble, but the way he pretended made us all smile.

After about five minutes, Mom said she had to go. She told Noah she was going to make some dinner and then go to bed early. Noah kissed the phone as he said goodbye.

"I love you guys," Mom said.

With the unthinking ease of having said it a million times before, I replied:

"I love you, goodbye."

WE WOKE up early the next day, just after sunrise, to bright morning light streaming into our east-facing apartment. We sat on the little red couch in the living room and talked about how we needed to get out of the house, for Noah's sake, despite the fact that we were both still sad over losing our pet.

Then Rebekah's phone rang.

Her phone had been connected to her iPad, so when it rang, we could answer the call on either device. As we browsed the iPad for something fun to do on Canada Day, the call screen popped up. We weren't immediately sure where her phone was, so I tapped the screen on the iPad to answer the call. It seemed there was a lot happening all at once. I was a little irritated that someone would be calling us so early in the morning.

It was my sister's husband, Shaun. He didn't say hello. "I'm sorry to tell you," he started. He stopped, took a breath, then continued. "Your mom passed away last night."

I felt my heart beat hard in my chest, exactly six times.

Thump, thump, thump, thump, thump, thump.

Then the sounds stopped. My whole world stopped. I heard the words, but they didn't make sense.

In that moment, my brain interpreted it as a cruel joke. "Hang up the fucking phone," I snapped. "That fucking asshole." Shaun

254

was a prankster. My gullible mother was often on the receiving end of his jokes. However, the death of my mother was off limits. It wasn't funny. She can't die. She won't die. Not now, not ever— that's not part of the plan.

Rebekah managed to fumble around with the iPad and switch the call over to her phone. I watched her face, still, darkening, through a haze. She handed the phone back to me. Shaun put my sister on the line. When I heard her voice, that's when I understood. This wasn't a joke.

My mother was dead.

My sister could hardly speak. I was having trouble processing her words anyway. They were next door to Mom's apartment, at what we still thought of as my grandmother's, where Nana Ag had raised my mother and most of her family. A few family members had started to gather. By noon, we knew, the place would be packed.

My sister told me that Mom had been found less than an hour earlier. Gary came to pick her up for an early breakfast, and he was the one who found her. She was in her bathtub. The paramedics were still on the scene and her body was still there. From the preliminary information they had so far, rigor mortis had set in. She'd been dead for several hours. She had died before sunrise.

She was naked, but the bathtub was empty. It was as though she got up around three in the morning to take a bath, as she sometimes did when she couldn't sleep, but forgot to fill the tub with water. There were no signs of struggle, nothing out of place, no injuries. We were told that she was slumped over but otherwise looked peaceful. We immediately assumed that she'd had another massive seizure, or a stroke, or a heart attack, but nobody knew for sure.

"Does Raymond know yet?" I asked Krista.

"No, I couldn't get a hold of him," she said.

"Okay, I'll try to reach him," I answered.

There was a mix of voices in the background. The phone was muffled under my sister's hand, but I heard her ask someone what was happening. She came back on the line.

"I think they're taking Mom's body out now," she said. "They're taking her away. I have to go."

"Okay," I said, detaching. "I'll try to reach Raymond and I'll call back in a little while."

I hung up and called my brother. No answer. I texted him: "Ray, call me as soon as you get this. It's an emergency."

Within minutes, my phone rang. I could hear my brother speaking to someone else as I answered. "Hang on, he said it's an emergency! Hello?"

"Hey, um, are you somewhere private right now?" I don't know why that mattered.

"Yeah, what's up?" he asked with his usual impatience.

"It's Mom," I said.

He made a sound, a cracking gasp.

I could hear his tears before I even said it. Miles and years and personalities apart, siblings still share worst fears.

"What's wrong?" he asked. He said it as if he already knew but wished he didn't.

"Ray, she's dead."

The line went silent.

It seemed like an eternity. I didn't know what else to say.

"What happened?" he finally asked. His voice was thick with confusion and denial.

"She had a seizure last night," I said. I didn't have any idea if that was true, but it was an easy explanation. "Ray, she's gone," I said. That was true.

Raymond became overwhelmed. "I have to go," he said, and the line disconnected.

The room was quiet, whatever room I was in, wherever I was. I didn't know. My mind was spinning. I kept expecting myself to wake up, but I knew I wouldn't. I suddenly realized that I had to get back home.

I dragged out my laptop and began hammering half-blind at the keys. There were only two options to get to Sydney direct, and neither would get me there very quickly. And I had another problem: I didn't have any money. Money wasn't something that just sat around in my bank account waiting for an emergency. Each and every month, it came in and went back out to pay the rent and bills.

I racked my brain for somebody who might be able to help. My boss came to mind. She and I had developed a close relationship in my short time working for her. I called her at her office. I don't remember how she figured out what was going on, because I just kept repeating myself over and over.

"I have to go home," I said. "I have to go home. I have to go home."

Rebekah took the phone from my hands. I could feel myself shaking all over. My skin was cold and clammy. I was breathing fast and shallow. My eyes darted around, looking for nothing, hoping for something. I was suddenly having a panic attack.

Rebekah guided me into our bedroom, where I made my way to the bed. I lay down on top of the sheets with my arms by my sides, stiff and cold. I stared up at the ceiling. I didn't fall asleep, at least not in the usual sense. But the world seemed to fade away.

Sometime later—I'm not sure how long I was in that trance—Rebekah came back in. She told me she had spoken to my boss and that she was going to arrange and pay for our flights home. The departure time was later that day. I had no idea what to do until then.

There was a knock at the front door, and Rebekah went to answer it. I got up from the bed and hovered nearby, feeling as if I was outside my body, watching the scenes before me unfold. Noah's nanny, Erin, was at the door. Rebekah had called her to come and care for Noah so that we could deal with the crisis at hand. I remember seeing her at the door, and the sad expression on her face, but the memory is thin.

After Noah was gone, and I was marginally more lucid, we decided that we couldn't possibly sit around at home for all the hours it would take before we had to go to the airport. Without anywhere in particular to go, we went to the car and drove. We went down the street a short way, turned a few times and ended up in a parking lot somewhere. We sat there in silence for at least an hour. Rebekah, always the pragmatist, eventually spoke up.

"Noah needs a white shirt," she said.

I had no idea how she could think about shopping at a time like this. Nothing made sense.

"Do you want me to pack your black suit for you?" she asked.

"What?" I said. "Why?"

She simply waited, looking at me gently. Then I realized that she was planning for my mother's funeral. I hadn't thought of that.

"Yes," I whispered.

I started the car and pulled away. We drove, mostly on auto-pilot, to the mall. I followed Rebekah around as she browsed the children's stores for a white shirt suitable for a toddler at a funeral. I still wasn't convinced that it mattered. She found one at the Gap, a simple white onesie with a collar and button-down front. As I watched her, feeling detached, I realized that she was detached too. The shopping was a distraction. I wondered if, of all the strangers who bustled around us, any of them could see our pain.

We spent the next few hours like this, distancing ourselves from time and reality as much as possible. My boss had called back to say she would drive us to the airport, so we made our way back to our apartment to pack. When she arrived, she awkwardly offered her condolences. She was broadsided by my trauma. Was it that obvious? It must have been.

We arrived at Pearson International in Toronto and somehow made it to our flight. I don't remember being in the airport. We had a layover of a few hours in Halifax, but it already seemed like the longest trip I'd ever taken anyway, so it was bearable. Noah enjoyed himself in a small play area, as unaware as you would expect a nearly two-year-old to be, while Rebekah and I looked on. We were called to our connecting flight and embarked on the final leg of our trip.

When we landed in Sydney about an hour later, Krista and Raymond met us at the airport. The moment my sister saw me, she collapsed in tears. My brother joined in, wrapping his arms around both of us in the uncomfortably tight way that he does. We stood there together, in the middle of a buzzing airport crowd, three newly un-mothered kids. As people around us looked on, we clung to each other, desperate, confused. My sister was soft, my brother felt rigid. I'm not sure what I was, or how I fit between them. I was somewhere between alive and dead, yesterday and today and tomorrow. It was purgatory.

I think I cried, but I don't remember. The fog rolled in.

The fog was a comfort.

CHAPTER 20

B Y THE TIME I GOT HOME TO CAPE BRETON, MOM'S body had been transported five hours away to Halifax for an autopsy. It was the same trip she'd taken with me in the back of an ambulance.

We went next door to Nana Ag's house. I guess it was Aunt Mary's house now, since Nana Ag was dead, but that didn't sound right. Life moves on in pieces. When we went in, the house, normally a place of laughter and joy, was instead filled with anguish. Mary was lost. Mom was her sister, but also her best friend. More family members arrived. Soon the kitchen would once more be full, as it often was over the years. As it was every Saturday night decades ago, when the Costigan family would clutch their rosaries and fall to their knees to pray. They were still praying, after all these years.

I went over to Mom's place to look around. Everything was exactly as it had been when I left at the end of March, and pretty much as she had always kept it. Her jacket was hanging on the hook by the door, her shoes on the floor beneath it. Her phone charger was on the arm of the couch, where I could picture her sitting with her feet up, playing whichever online game she sent me countless invitations to play with her. I wish I had played more often.

I went up the narrow staircase to the second floor. The whole unit was a mirror version of my grandmother's apartment. Mom's bedroom was the first on the right. The sheets had been turned down and her head print was still in the pillow. There was another bedroom across from hers that she sometimes used when she had company, like the last Christmas that Rebekah, Noah and I stayed with her. Down the hall, on the left, I went in her tiny bathroom. Her brush, glasses and cellphone were still sitting on the small counter by the sink. Everything was so neat. That was typical of Mom. I looked up at the medicine cabinet mirror above the sink and hardly recognized my own reflection. When did I get so many grey hairs? It had only been a day. Losing a parent changes you in an instant.

I approached the bathtub, knowing that's where she had died.

An image barged into my mind of her dead body lying there, stiff, grey and cold. Something didn't make sense. There was no suggestion from anyone of foul play, but I was trying to under-stand, because things like that aren't supposed to happen for no reason. She was found naked in the bathtub, but there was no water in the tub, or outside the tub either. There was no indica-tion that she had passed out and drowned. The investigator who attended the scene didn't think she had run the water at all. Then why would she get in? She always ran the water first, then got in, as most people would.

"I need to figure this out," I thought. If I figure it out, I can fix it.

The investigator said she had no injuries such as would result from a fall. There was also nothing at all out of place outside, inside or around the tub. The shower curtain was intact and the bottles in the corners hadn't been disturbed. If she had convulsed with another grand mal seizure, it must have happened after she got in and lay down, and it must have been very contained. He said that she was simply seated, slumped over, and that was it.

There were no clothes in the bathroom. Nothing discarded onto the floor after she undressed, nothing folded and ready for her to get out. Mom was not the type of person to walk around her house naked. She was too shy and self-conscious for that, even when alone. I remembered the white pyjamas she was wearing the last time I saw her alive.

I analyzed every last detail of every part of that bathroom.

I was looking for the mistake. Maybe it was all a big misunderstanding. It wasn't supposed to be this way, it wasn't right, it wasn't the plan. Maybe if I solved the problem of my mother's death, she wouldn't be dead anymore. Maybe I could resurrect her.

You are not the Christ.

I went back out into the L-shaped hallway and walked toward the third bedroom at the end. There was a red suitcase lying on top of the double bed, neatly packed with Mom's clothes. I looked through it carefully and recognized every piece. The clothes were mostly casual, as was Mom's style, but there was one dress. It was one of the two dresses she bought to wear to my wedding, the one that she liked better but didn't wear. There were gift certificates on her dresser for Inverary Resort, a peaceful getaway in Baddeck, Cape Breton. She and Gary were planning to take a short trip there the day she died, so she had packed the night before. Not long after she died, the historic resort burned to the ground. Fall, or be felled.

I retraced my steps, looking in each room again, going over and over the reconstruction of what might have happened. I went back downstairs. Her car was still parked outside. It was as though she had just run next door for a few minutes. Everything was so tidy, so normal. Normal catastrophe. Everyday catastrophe. A campfire isn't a catastrophe, but it contains all the necessary potential. Normal can be a catastrophe.

I stopped at the door before leaving. Almost without thinking, I buried my face in her jacket hanging on the hook nearby. It smelled just like her.

"You know that we'll always have each other, right?" she had said.

THE FIRST night back, we stayed with Rebekah's grandmother.

Gary came to visit us. I was sitting on the front step, alone, when he pulled up. He opened the door and hoisted himself out of the driver's seat in the same forceful way he always did. He was ten years older than my mother. She worried what would happen to her when he died. She fully expected he'd die first.

As he walked toward me, I was flooded with a lifetime of memories. He'd made us feel worthless, replaceable and weak for twenty years.

Be a man.

I don't think he even knew what he did to us. He seemed to think that he did us all a favour, that he'd saved us, redeemed us, as though we were the broken ones. As though we were the ones left shattered and alone.

As he walked toward me, he stumbled to the right, just a little.

He stopped. I'd been looking at his clenched fists as he walked toward me. I raised my eyes to his face. I felt a sharp breath catch in my throat.

He was broken. There was no mistaking it. You know a shattered man when you see one. In that moment, we had everything in common.

I got up and stepped forward as he closed the distance between us. As he got within about ten feet, he raised his fists like he was getting ready for a fight. He was a tough guy, a man's man, a fighter. This time was different. He couldn't fight his way out of this any more than I could figure it out. This was a fight he'd already lost, and a problem I couldn't solve.

His nine meaty fingers released from his calloused palms. His hands stretched out. I don't know if he was reaching out for me in front of him or pleading to God above him.

For the first time, he came directly to me. He wrapped his arms around me, weak and clumsy. His face slack, he cried. He cried hard, loud and blind. He pawed at me, helpless, as if he didn't know what to do with his body. I don't know if Gary had the capacity for a sensitive emotion like sadness. I'd never seen him cry before. I think his tears were pain. He knew pain.

I'd known Gary for more than twenty years, but I think this was the first time I truly saw him. He was flawed. He had said and done things to us over the years that I didn't know if I could ever forgive. But in this moment, he was human. He was stripped bare and broken. He was just like me.

That first night spent with the knowledge that my mom was no longer somewhere in the world, that I could no longer pick up the phone and call her at any time, was one of the longest nights of my life. I'd come a long way, but I wasn't ready to not be mothered anymore. I didn't yet trust my ability to walk on my own, to lead a life without my mom. I tossed and turned in the uncomfortable double bed all night, finding new complaints: It's too cold. The dog is bothering my allergies. The street light outside is too bright.

Really, I couldn't close my eyes. I was afraid. That first night was when the nightmares started. They came every night after that for months. Sometimes the nightmares would even creep in during waking hours, at quiet or stressful or random moments during the day.

Each time it was the same.

Every time I closed my eyes, I saw my mother's dead body lying naked on an autopsy table, her face peeled down over her nose, her skull sawed open.

MOM WAS sent back home without her brain.

The medical examiner was not able to determine a definitive cause of death and kept her brain for further analysis. Mom would have joked about her forgetfulness in her self-deprecating way by saying she had left her brain somewhere. Mom would have appreciated the irony, in this fictional world of our minds in which she was still alive, a desperate creation of our coping imaginations. What else could we do?

All the business and event planning involved with death happened in the fog. We arranged the priest and the funeral mass. I was going to speak before the funeral, as I had at my grandmother's. We visited the funeral home and picked out a casket—a pretty, glossy white one with little rose details. Mom would have liked that. We made these kinds of guesses a lot, thinking about what Mom would have liked. Everybody seemed to know her a little differently. Each of us remembered her as we needed to.

Gary honestly seemed to think he was my mother's hero. That's what he needed to believe. He was adamant that the obituary be a fawning ode to Mom's love for him, "the love of her life," as he insisted that he be called. A few of us knew that only weeks before she died, she had thrown the decades-old engagement ring back at Gary, as she had a few times in the past. Mom later spotted the ring on the finger of Little Gary's girlfriend. My mother was so upset, even though she had thrown it back at him, that Gary could just give the ring away for his son to recycle on someone else. It reinforced for her that the ring wasn't a promise of love; it was a symbol of ownership. Mom didn't want to be owned anymore. The happiest and most confident I ever saw her had been in the last few years, when she was finally living independently and having a relationship on her own terms. She had transformed.

Krista and I were inseparable during this time. We balanced each other well. Her emotions were all over the place, while I tried to maintain a cool, reasonable detachment. Raymond was different. He had been on his own for years, and had never really seemed to move on, more or less, the way the rest of us did. Mom and I argued more than once about how I felt she enabled him to live in a narrative that life happened to him, that he never had any opportunities, that he was a victim of every injustice.

As we were preparing for the wake, Rebekah and I went back to Mom's house to find her something to wear. We picked the dress that she had packed for her trip. So, really, my mom had picked her own outfit; she was just taking a different sort of trip than she had planned. I went to the bathroom to get her glasses from the counter, but they were gone. Her cellphone was still there, and the brush too, but her glasses were gone. I went to her bedroom to find the cross that she usually wore around her neck. It was gone too. I opened her jewellery box and it was a tangled mess, which was very uncharacteristic of Mom. It looked as though the jewellery box had been dumped out, rummaged through and dumped back.

There were other items missing from her room too, including jewellery, clothes and sentimental trinkets. Mom didn't have anything of much value, so it all seemed very arbitrary. My sister and I knew it must've been our brother. It seemed like something Raymond would do. He denied it, for a while, before some items were eventually returned. We all deal with shock and grief differently, often falling back on familiar coping mechanisms. Maybe Ray unconsciously thought he could steal Mom back to life. As someone who wanted to think her back to life, I couldn't hold that against him. He eventually told me that he blindly grabbed armfuls of random things: eyeglasses, cheap jewellery, clothes, a pair of her shoes. He kept the shoes near the front door of his house for three years. Every time he saw them, he said, it made him feel like she was there with him.

I collected an older pair of glasses, a different cross and a set of earrings that she liked and put them with the dress. Rebekah was in charge of her undergarments—I didn't want to do that. We brought everything to the funeral home.

At the wake the next day, Gary wanted to approach the casket first. I encouraged everyone to agree, that it wasn't a big deal, so we could avoid confrontation. "Blessed are the peacemakers," I thought. Part of me just didn't think it made much of a difference.

After a short period of time—which Krista would later complain was much longer—the rest of us approached the casket too. The remains in the casket looked enough like my mother that she was recognizable. It looked like her, but it wasn't her. It was what was left of her. Krista was unhappy that Mom appeared to her to be frowning, so the funeral director adjusted her expression between visitations. If only we were all so fortunate, I thought, to be fixed so easily.

The priest from Holy Redeemer arrived. Priests at Holy Redeemer didn't change very often; there weren't enough to choose from. But everything changes eventually, given enough time. This was not the priest with whom I served as an altar boy for so many years, who had prayed over my comatose body in the hospital.

"May the Lord, who frees you from sin, save you and raise you up," he said.

Father Errol had died on Christmas Day. The new pastor was Father Murphy. He was the same priest who had married Rebekah and me, and who baptized Noah. He said that, since Mom had died so suddenly, without the benefit of the prayers of last rites, he would pray for her soul. I felt my body tense. I'd forgotten about that. He opened one of the familiar-looking texts and read. He got to the part about forgiveness.

"God of love," he said, "welcome your daughter Brenda, whom you have called from this life. Release her from all her sins, bless her with eternal light and peace, raise her up to live forever . . ."

I felt a rush of relief that I hadn't realized I was anticipating. Faith, especially Catholicism, had played an important part in my upbringing. It was always in the background, and even if I never really thought myself very good at it, it provided me with routine, comfort, hope. But it cracked. How could God let this happen?

The wake, for me, had all the significance of a few hundred people filing dutifully through a building to look at an old hat that someone had left behind. Ritual used to give me comfort because I always knew exactly what to expect. Now it felt hollow. Everything seemed so procedural.

"It's just procedure," I recalled one of the anonymous nurses saying to me as I lay restrained on the stretcher in the psych ward as a kid. Just another procedural trauma.

My sister and I stood at our post near Mom's feet. We stood there for an hour or so each day, for two days, greeting and thanking the long line of people as they walked by. It was exhausting. My brother stood with us for the first few people, but staying in one place for longer than a few minutes had never been Ray's thing. We understood. We greeted the line of people who came to pay their respects. There were hundreds of them, at least half of whom, it seemed, were anonymous nurses. They all seemed to know us. Mom had talked about us a lot.

During the wake and funeral, glimpses of Gary's habitual self started to come back. Personalities, like statistics, have a powerful tendency to revert to the mean. They go back to whatever their normal is. Rather than stand with us, he planted himself about ten feet away, talking to people before they got to us. More than a few of them looked uncomfortable at how long he held them hostage. Had they experienced Gary's sermons as I did, I thought, they would have known that they couldn't just leave. That's not how hostage situations work. My mother's death made me think a lot about my childhood experiences. Grieving her finally forced me to also grieve and eventually accept that entire time in my life too. Now it's over.

I was the last one to spend some private time with what was left of my mother before the casket was closed and transported to the church. Holy Redeemer was right across the street. Mom was born, married, divorced and died within a few square kilometres of the church. That's how life in a small town was supposed to go.

I knelt by her side and talked to her, trying to force myself to find a connection to the moment I'd been avoiding. I sang her a few verses of an old Irish folk song, "A Mother's Love Is a Blessing." Father Errol used to sing it every Mother's Day in church, and Mom loved it. She sent me videos of it a few times over the years.

A mother's love is a blessing, no matter where you roam.
Love her while she's living, for you'll miss her when she's gone.
Love her as in childhood, when feeble, old and grey,
For you'll never miss a mother's love, till she's buried beneath
the clay.

I still felt detached at the funeral. It all seemed silly, all these people, all these words and songs and ceremonies, smells and bells, all for a box occupied by a body, an empty human, a former mother. It was just like Mom's memory box, filled with inanimate objects enlivened by the memories they trigger.

"That's not my mom in that box," I thought. "There's nothing at all in that box. Just a reminder."

I said a few words from the lectern to the gathered masses before the funeral started, something about love, and sang that Irish folk song for the first and last time. Then I sat and watched the proceedings. When the mass was ending, and the pallbearers were preparing to wheel my mother outside to the waiting hearse, I felt an incredible urge to throw myself into the aisle. I wanted to scream. I wanted to tell them, No, you can't take my mom away. I won't let you. I'm not ready.

They did, and I followed.

I went to the cemetery in one of the funeral home limousines with their four-way flashers on. Cape Breton was still a place where people pulled to the side of the road for a passing funeral procession. I never saw that happen in Toronto, but I always pulled over. Habits are hard to kill. We got to Resurrection Cemetery, where I'd been visiting my grandfather's grave since I was a little kid, every November on All Souls' Day. It was where my grandmother had recently been buried beside him. It was the final resting place of a handful of other family members as well. The plot we bought for my mother was a row or two down from her mother's. She was buried on a grassy hill overlooking a big lake, which I thought was just about the most peaceful place on Earth.

Gary initially wouldn't pay anything toward any of the funeral or burial expenses. I did a lot of badgering, just as I'd done when I lost the game of Trouble when I was twelve. He finally made a contribution, a small fraction of the total expense, leaving the rest to be split three ways between my sister, brother and me. Mom had left him her entire pension, changing her policy to make him the beneficiary only a few months before she died. That guaranteed Gary would be paid the remainder of the principal amount that Mom never got to use in retirement. The insurance company decided to grant Gary a lifetime payment as well, because of his relationship with Mom. It apparently didn't matter that they hadn't lived together in years and were no longer engaged. "We read the obituary," the lady from the company said on the phone, informing us of the details. It was the obituary that I wrote, with Gary at my shoulder, describing him as the love of my mother's life. None of that sat well with Krista or Raymond, but I tried my best to keep the peace.

Mom named me, my sister and my brother as beneficiaries of a modest new life insurance policy acquired around the same time she made Gary her pension beneficiary in place of us. We wondered if Mom had known something about her health that we didn't. Ray said that Mom had confessed everything to him. We knew that she didn't, because according to her doctor there was nothing to tell. Raymond wanted to feel special. We all did. Krista wondered if whatever was happening in our mother's brain had impaired her decision-making. Before and after her death, nothing made any sense.

The morning after the funeral, Rebekah and I went back down to Mom's apartment to start taking stock of what needed to be done. The death cleaning. When we pulled around the corner at about eight o'clock, we saw that Mom's door was propped open. Two of her sisters, Peggy and Marie, were carrying furniture and boxes out to their cars. I parked quickly and rushed toward them.

"What are you doing?" I asked Peggy urgently when she came back out.

"Gary told us to clear everything out," she replied.

"You can't do that. You have to put everything back." I was panicked.

"What?" Marie was there now. "What's going on?"

"Oh my god," I said. "Krista is going to lose her mind." I couldn't believe what was happening. "You have to put everything back the way you found it. Krista hasn't even been down to go through everything yet. You have to put everything back."

"I'm sorry," Peggy answered, almost in tears. "I'm sorry, we didn't know. Gary said to do it. He told us to come down and get everything out fast."

When Gary had a job to do, he'd get it done well, but he liked to get it done fast. This was the same person who moved us out of our house on Lingan Road in a day, who renovated his basement so many times, and who was constantly retreating from a world he didn't understand by landscaping his property at the bottom of the dead-end dirt road from sunrise to well after nightfall. But I wasn't about to let him erase my mother that quickly. I needed more time—we all did—to adapt to this life-altering change.

Gary generally avoided me and my sister after the funeral. I had two more calls with him, checking in to see if he was doing okay. Then he started screening and avoiding my calls. I knew he was, because when I tried calling from an unlisted number, he answered. Then his son Gary Jr. started to answer instead. He'd end the call quickly by saying that his father wasn't home or didn't want to talk. Gary had finally got all The Henicks out of his life after all, I thought. I was hurt. I didn't want to be. I hated that I was. I didn't want him to matter. But he did.

Sometimes we can't control who matters to us.

Losing my mother was the single most traumatic experience of my life. Everything that happened after her death only compounded the trauma. But there was something different this time. I'd been preparing all my life for this moment. I would need everything I'd been through and learned to get through this—everything I didn't ask for, every mistake and struggle, every success and beautiful, hopeful milestone. I would need to call upon every part of myself. It will be hard. Life is hard.

In the week following her funeral, Rebekah, my sister and I gradually cleared everything out of Mom's apartment. As I was leaving for the final time, I remembered the last time I'd hugged her, and how she waved from this same door. I remembered her tears, the unexpected lump in my throat.

"It's not weird to love your mother," I thought.

"A mother's love is a blessing," I sang.

I stopped outside Mom's vacant apartment. I looked left, to Nana Ag's place next door. I looked beyond it, up the street to where I had ridden my purple bicycle, and I followed it in my imagination, screaming down Railroad Street. From Mom's front step I looked right, toward the overpass, the shadow it cast on the ground below. It looked small from down here.

274

Everything did. It's funny, when you grow up, how things look smaller than they did when you were little. Sometimes you don't realize how far you've come until you stop and look back. I'd come so far.

The July sun, for a moment, broke through the rain clouds. I looked up and felt the sun on my face. It reminded me that, even though rain falls and the seasons change, summer always returns. But not yet. I broke down and cried. Rebekah held my hand, as she had done so many times since we were sixteen. She squeezed, a reminder that she was there for me, that we had each other. I squeezed back. I hadn't forgotten. Sometimes all you can do is hold hands.

"Nothing will ever be the same," I said through my tears. "This changes everything."

"It does," she agreed. She didn't say anything else. There were no more comforting words, or rationalizations, or profound revelations. It was just a fact. Everything would be different now, and there was nothing I could do about it. Nothing, that is, except eventually learn to accept it and move on.

Nothing changes if nothing changes.

All this time, I thought I'd been recovering. Ever since the man on the bridge saved me, I'd really just been running. My whole life had been a desperate attempt to escape. But I couldn't run from this. I couldn't escape death. What I could do, however, was cherish the time I had. Although I didn't know how long I had left, I finally felt as though I would have plenty of time to be dead later. Until then, I'll live, and struggle, and love, and suffer, and grow. My recovery was just getting started.

I took a moment, then turned back to pull the door to Mom's apartment closed. Before I did, I looked inside. In my mother's empty living room, I finally saw the end of my childhood, such as it was. I saw my identity as a son, "the baby," as Mom's friends all called me, the hopeless case—it all came to its conclusion.

As I pulled the door closed, Mom's voice echoed in my mind. I heard her last words to me and my new family, as we started our new life.

I love you, she said.

I answered my mother once more, with the ease of having said it a million times before.

"I love you, goodbye."

Epilogue

"DADDY, ARE YOU GOING TO DIE?"

My son Noah's big brown eyes looked up at me with curious concern. I wasn't surprised by the question. He'd been surrounded by death since my mom died just before his second birthday. As I looked at the six-year-old lying in his bed next to me, it seemed like a lifetime ago. I felt guilty about the grief that he grew up with. I'd always planned for him to know a happier life than me, maybe even a perfect one. Then, well, life happened. Life was hard, but I kept choosing to do it anyway.

Noah talked about my mom often, probably because I talked to him about her so much in the year or two after she died. Every night before bed, in fact, I reminded him that his Nana Brenda was watching over him from heaven. I'm not sure how much I believed that—I'd lost a lot of faith after she died—but sometimes habits are hard to kill. I'm not sure how much he remembered of her, either. Still, I reflected on how it's not the things we remember that define us, but the stories we tell ourselves about the things we think we remember.

Meanwhile, Noah continued to watch me steadily. He'd become a grounding force for me. He could pull me back from my thoughts with his way of always being in the present moment.

"Daddy," he insisted. "Are you going to die?"

"Not for a very long time, Noah," I said.

"Will you still be alive when I'm a daddy too?"

I thought for a minute.

"I hope so," I answered. I realized that I really, really did. I looked forward to it.

He asked me to scratch his back, in the tickly way that he liked, which I also liked when I was his age. He fell asleep. I kissed his head and tucked him in.

"Tuck, tuck, tuck," I whispered instinctively, the way my dad did, as I tightened the blankets around him. I left his room and stopped outside the door.

"One down," I sighed to myself. The beauty of parenting is exhausting, I was learning.

I made my way to the kitchen and grabbed the bottle on the counter that had already been prepared. You figure out the rhythm and shortcuts of parenting after a while. Time can make the hard stuff a little easier. I took it to Theodore, Noah's younger brother, who was standing and waiting in his crib. He looked a lot more like me than Noah but was much more grounded, like my wife. Noah is brilliant, creative, emotional. Theo is funny, secure, a little brash. Each of them is exactly the brother that the other needs. I picked him up and brought him to the rocking chair that we bought when we had Noah. He cuddled in and we read from Julia Donaldson's classic, *The Gruffalo*.

I read in a quiet, animated voice, one more confident in being a dad than it was the first time I read this book. Being a parent didn't scare me as much anymore. With time, and mistakes, and beautiful, rare victories, you learn, you grow, you spiral up. I'm grateful to have learned that from my worst moments. Otherwise, my best moments might have passed me by uncherished. "All was quiet, in the deep dark wood," I read. "The mouse found a nut and the nut was good."

"One more?" Theodore asked, as I expected he would.

"I love you, Theo," I replied. "Mommy and Noah love you too." I didn't add that Nana Brenda loved him in his nightly script, even if I knew it somewhere in my heart to be a post-mortem truth. I was so anxious to have a second child after my mom died. She'd never know him. If my life moved on without her, it would confirm that she was, indeed, dead. Life moved on anyway. I discovered ever newer parts of myself as it did, in a way I never thought possible in my resistance to letting go. It was good.

I gave him his bottle, turned out the lights and left his room. "Two down," I muttered to myself.

I checked in on my wife. My high school sweetheart, whom I've been with since only a few months after Mike saved my life. She was asleep in our bedroom, lying in bed with Adeline, our daughter. She was born just before Theo turned two. She looks like Theo but has Noah's personality. That is, she's tough and creative. We named her Adeline Brenda Carol, after my mom, and every time I look at her, I see my entire maternal lineage in her soft face. She was asleep in my sleeping wife's arms. I stroked her cheek and quietly retreated to my desk, to continue working on my long-suffering memoir.

After finding Mike, I had become increasingly dissatisfied with climbing the professional ladder. I quit my job shortly after I was asked to write this book. I decided to run toward that change rather than away, with more enthusiasm than I'd ever had before. I decided that life was far too short to do anything except what I was most passionate about. For me, that was speaking to audiences and writing alone, oscillating between two worlds of silence and of sound, so that's what I did now. The writing especially gave me a lot of time to think; it demanded it of me.

I thought about the steel plant in Sydney. I had spent a lot of time there, in my mind, while writing this memoir. I revisited every square inch of it. In reality, too, I had gone back there, to measure the distance of my intended fall, to talk with the people who knew me and that place, to pick up the boxes of medical records and police reports I drew upon in piecing together this story as best I could. It was a park now, grassy and serene, buzzing with families, the kids young enough that they had never known what the place used to be. Nothing changes if nothing changes, but eventually, something changes everything. Sometimes things change right under your nose and you don't realize until you've got enough distance. Nana Ag is gone now, but her backyard, where everything was painted the same flaking shade of grey, is still visible from the overpass.

When I stood on that edge of concrete all those years ago, looking out over that place I thought would never change, looking inside at my inner turmoil that I also thought was unchangeable, I didn't know who I was. I was helpless, I was hopeless.

I was convinced then that it was the end.

Now, I looked at my life. From the many misshapen and scattered stones of my childhood, I had finally built a house on rock. My mother always wanted to do what her mother did: to make a house a home, to fill it with memories and hope and faith. She wanted peace. She passed that desire on to me. There was much to do, but I would do the work. It wasn't perfect, but it was good. I finally felt good. I didn't need the safety of certainty anymore.

Whatever happens next, I have the only certainty I need, planted deep in my soul. I remind myself of it every time I encounter adversity great and small.

This is not the end.

ACKNOWLEDGEMENTS

Robert Mackwood at Seventh Avenue Literary Agency for seeing the potential in this from the very beginning.

Jim Gifford at HarperCollins Canada for his patience and steady hand in editing and publishing this work.

Janice Zawerbny at HarperCollins Canada for using fresh eyes to take the manuscript to the next level.

John Sweet, my copy editor, and Natalie Meditsky, my production editor, and all of those who worked behind the scenes to polish this stone.

The Trappist brothers of Calvary Abbey in Rogersville, New Brunswick, for providing a quiet place to be with my thoughts, and where I wrote and rewrote much of this book. There's a rock there with an inscription that I read every day: "He that shall endure unto the end, the same shall be saved. —Mk 13, 13."

The Trappist brothers of Genesee Abbey in Piffard, New York, for giving me the structure to persevere through the longer than expected editing process.

Jeanne-Marie Robillard at the National Speakers Bureau for her support in getting this project started.

Martin Perelmuter and Farah Perelmuter at Speakers' Spotlight for seeing and supporting the future of this project.

Rosie O'Donnell, I'm convinced that this book never would have gotten off the ground had it not been for your early acknowledgement, and ongoing support and encouragement. Your generosity and warmth made a mere mortal like me feel special, which is no small feat.

Rona Maynard, your early advice to stop "sounding so writerly" rang in my memory repeatedly. It reminded me to let down my wordy defences. Thank you for that, and for your early reading and comments.

Neil Pasricha for your ongoing encouragement and enthusiasm, especially in dedicating my whole self to this.

Dr. Brian Goldman for your notes, your advice to find my voice and your unwavering support.

Ann Douglas for your kindness and encouragement, your gentle spirit and inspiration.

Lesley Carew for talking me down with warmth and humour when I was convinced that everything about this project was going to hell.

Andrew Solomon for always taking the time to respond to me, and for sharing a little glimpse of your life. Your work has changed me, and has provided a model to which I aspire.

Tanya O'Brien, of Moncton, New Brunswick. I said I would thank you in the acknowledgements of my book way back in 2018 during Bell Let's Talk day. I'm a person of my word. Thank you for your support.

Those members of both the Costigan and Henick extended families who shared their own memories with me, especially since it wasn't always easy. A lot of it didn't make the final draft, but it informed every page, and it'll never be cut from my memory.

My sister, Krista Woodill, for her patience in answering my endless questions, and for her support of my family while I was absent in either body or mind.

My father, Shaun, and my brother, Raymond. We share so much more than blood alone.

Donnie Holland for saving my life the first time.

Mike Richey for saving my life the last time.

Rebekah, Noah, Theodore and Adeline for saving my life every day, for giving me life, for being my life. Thank you for supporting me on this wild, uncertain journey. Thank you for letting me love you. You redeem me. Thank you.